I0830833

INTERMITTENT FASTING

The ultimate guide to knowing and getting all the benefits of autophagy

Damon Reed

Galatea Publishing

Intermittent Fasting. The ultimate guide to knowing and getting all the benefits of autophagy, by Damon Reed.

TABLE OF CONTENTS

INTRODUCTION 11

THE PROBLEM OF OUR MODERN DIET 12

FOOD HAS THE NUTRIENTS YOU NEED, BUT CANNED OR PREPROCESSED FOODS DON'T. 12

SERIOUS ILLNESSES ARE OFTEN CAUSED BY A POOR DIET..................................13

COMPANIES REPLACE HARMFUL ADDITIVES WITH WORSE ONES 13

IT IS DIFFICULT TO FIND 100% HEALTHY FOOD 14

PROBLEM FOODS BEHIND THE CURRENT OBESITY EPIDEMIC 14

Corn puffs, among other packaged treats 15

Fried food...15

Energy drinks, sodas and bottled 'natural' juices..........................16

Biscuits and bread 16

Candies, cakes, desserts and jellies 17

WHAT IS THE MAIN PROBLEM WITH TODAY'S MEALS? 17

HISTORY OF INTERMITTENT FASTING 19

SCIENTIFIC FOUNDATIONS OF INTERMITTENT FASTING 22

WHAT IS HUNGER?...22

Is eating 6 times a day discouraged?..23

Is hunger really a mental problem? 23

Nipping 'mental hunger' in the bud 26

Can hunger be avoided while my body gets used to fasting? 27

Water as an ally in fasting..29

What are electrolytes and how can they help me reduce my hunger?.......30

The solution to alleviate hunger at the beginning of intermittent fasting ..30

Emotional hunger and how to identify it....................................30

DIFFERENCES BETWEEN REAL HUNGER, MENTAL HUNGER AND EMOTIONAL HUNGER 31

Emotional hunger 32

Mental hunger or for habit 32

Real hunger 32

WILL I BE HUNGRY WHEN I START FASTING? 33

WHAT HAPPENS TO OUR BODY WHEN WE FAST?.......................................34

What happens to the body if you fast for 12 hours? 34

What happens to the body after an ideal 16-hour fast?....................35

Fasting for several days and its advantages 35

What happens in the body with an interdaily fast?.........................36

ALL THE BENEFITS AND ADVANTAGES OF FASTING......................................37

Fasting helps end emotional hunger 37

Intermittent fasting increases and improves immune system functions.....38

Controlled fasting will help you lose weight and keep it off 38

Intermittent fasting will lower your blood sugar levels 39
Fasting will give your stomach and digestive system in general a rest. 40
Does it help you live longer? 40
It is a depurative method 41
Improve concentration for practicing various spiritual or functional
activities... 41
Improves the appearance of the skin 42
It saves you a good part of your income 42
Other benefits of intermittent fasting you need to know 42

THE RELATIONSHIP BETWEEN METABOLISM AND FASTING 44

METABOLIC PHASES OF FASTING.. 45
How long can the body tolerate fasting metabolically speaking?............. 46
Fasting and lost electrolytes 47
Other physiological phenomena occurring during fasting......................... 47

TYPES OF INTERMITTENT FASTING 49

TYPE 12/12 INTERMITTENT FASTING (TIME RESTRICTED FEEDING) 49
16/8 INTERMITTENT FASTING: THE STARTING POINT FOR A HEALTHY LIFE 51
EAT-STOP-EAT INTERMITTENT FASTING 51
SEMI-FASTING TYPE INTERMITTENT FASTING (FASTING MIMICKING DIET) 52
5:2 FASTING 52
THE WARRIOR DIET.. 53
Is the Warrior Diet really worth it? 54
24-HOUR INTERMITTENT FASTING 55

WHAT CAN YOU DRINK DURING YOUR FAST? 56

DRINKS YOU CAN HAVE DURING INTERMITTENT FASTING 56
Infusions 56
Sodas with low or no sugar content 59
THE IMPORTANCE OF HYDRATING WITH WATER 59

DIABETES AND INTERMITTENT FASTING: COMPATIBLE? 61

INTERMITTENT FASTING AND TYPE 1 DIABETES... 62
INTERMITTENT FASTING AND TYPE 2 DIABETES... 63
ADVANTAGES OF INTERMITTENT FASTING WITH TYPE 2 DIABETES 63
You won't have to count calories 64
It is effective in controlling blood sugar levels 64
DANGERS OR DISADVANTAGES OF INTERMITTENT FASTING WITH TYPE 2 DIABETES 65
There is a lack of glycemic control 65
The process of adapting to intermittent fasting will be more difficult 65
You may feel a bigger appetite and eat more during your next meal......... 66
CAN INTERMITTENT FASTING HELP IN CASE OF DIABETES RISK? 66
REASONS WHY INTERMITTENT FASTING WORKS FOR TYPE 2 DIABETES............ 67

FASTING AND THE BRAIN..**69**

Evolution, Intermittent Fasting, and the Brain...69

FASTING AND THE HEART..**71**

Surprise! Bad cholesterol does not solely depend on nutrition.....................72
Intermittent fasting as a definitive method for lowering cholesterol 74

FASTING AND EXERCISE..**76**

The body and its energy system 77
Can I combine intermittent fasting with exercise to lose weight?.................79
When is it best to exercise while fasting? 80
Essential food when you exercise while fasting 80
Contraindications when fasting and practicing sports 82

INTERMITTENT FASTING IN WOMEN **83**

Is intermittent fasting healthy on a hormonal level for women?...................83
Should I avoid intermittent fasting as a woman? 84
So, should women fast?...87

MEN AND INTERMITTENT FASTING..**88**

What if I am not interested in gaining muscle but in losing weight?.............89
Intermittent fasting and testosterone: you should increase your levels..........89

FOODS TO EAT AFTER THE FASTING PERIOD (AND BREAKING IT) **90**

Hydration is vital 90
Breaking the fast with solid foods gradually..91
Types of Foods That Work Great for Breaking the Fast 91
Foods and drinks that you should not consider to break the fast 92
What happens if I accidentally drink alcohol to break my fast?...................92
Refeeding syndrome after fasting..92
Risk factors for Refeeding syndrome 93
How do you avoid refeeding syndrome after heavy fasting? 94

TIPS TO ADOPT INTERMITTENT FASTING IN YOUR LIFE **95**

Choose the right fasting plan..95
Don't rush, your body will let you know when it's ready 96
Get used to doing everything in stages..96
The detox phase 97
The high protein and high fat phase 97
The hydrate phase 98
In the variety lies the secret..98
Drink liquids to replace meals 99
Eat your last meal of the day in the late afternoon.......................................99

FAILURE IS HUMAN 100

MAKE COMFORT PREVAIL 101

MYTH 1. STOP EATING FOR A DAY? IMPOSSIBLE! 102

MYTH 2. FASTING WILL CAUSE THE BODY TO RECEIVE FEWER NUTRIENTS! 103

MYTH 3. FASTING LEADS TO THE NEED TO EAT MORE AFTERWARDS 103

MYTH 4. FASTING CAUSES LOW BLOOD SUGAR LEVELS 104

WHO SHOULD NOT FAST?.. 106

Nursing mothers 106

Pregnant women... 106

Complications of type 1 diabetes 107

You are very underweight 107

Children and teenagers 108

People suffering from reflux disease (GERD) 108

CONCLUSIONS 109

BIBLIOGRAPHY 111

INTERMITTENT FASTING

The ultimate guide to knowing and getting all the benefits of autophagy

Damon Reed

Galatea Publishing

Introduction

Throughout the centuries we have seen how different cultures and religions use fasting as a purifying method, either for the spirit or for the health of the body. Today, fasting is very different from starvation, since in the first case certain foods are forbidden to the body in order to sacrifice something that we like very much, but that is bad for the body (or for spiritual purposes, as a method of sacrifice), while in the second case there is no certainty of when we will eat again after consuming a meal.

An example of spiritual fasting is found in the most significant book for Christians, the Bible, where Jesus Christ fasted for 40 days for spiritual purposes; not because he lacked food, but because he wanted to have a close relationship with God spiritually. However, starvation occurs when you do not know when you will eat next or what the next meal will be; an example is the starvation that occurred during the siege of Paris, in which the Parisians trapped in the city had no access to food, even if they wanted to eat. Fasting, on the other hand, is a voluntary practice whereby the body is deprived of certain types of food, although at any time it can be resumed at will. With **intermittent fasting**, the body can be deprived of foods with a high glycemic index on a daily basis, at certain times of the day, seasonally or for weeks, which represents not a diet, but a lifestyle to eat what we want and avoid gaining weight by doing so in full control. This book covers important aspects of intermittent fasting, so that you will recognize it as a powerful strategy to avoid obesity, high cholesterol, glucose, body fat and insulin. Welcome to the world of intermittent fasting!

CHAPTER I
The problem of our modern diet

The way we eat today is plagued with problems and deficiencies that silently attack our health. According to scientist Michael Polland, the current diet of a large majority of people has at least five major problems that must be addressed as soon as possible to avoid health problems and eating disorders. As a summary, here we have the five problems of modern eating that this wise scientist has studied over the years through studies.

Food has the nutrients you need, but canned or preprocessed foods don't.

It can seem very simple to cook an omelet and eat it with some special canned tuna, stocked with a large number of vegetables to add flavor to the mixture. However, there is a problem: these mass-produced food products have had a good part of their nutrients extracted so that they are preserved for months and the company insures its profits by preventing them from spoiling. The problem with these foods, therefore, is that although they can be prepared quickly (ideal for a busy lifestyle due to housework or work), they do not nourish you properly. In cases where vitamins and minerals are added artificially, they are still few compared to ones in fresh foods, as they never match the nutrients in their natural state. As if that were not enough, food companies brag about how these foods include added vitamins, proteins and minerals and that they increase the 'value' of their products, without making clear that it was the companies themselves who removed the natural nutrients initially present in these foods to begin with. This means that when you eat food of this type, especially canned ones, you are not eating in a healthy way, as you would with a good dish based on fresh food and ingredients, so be very careful with this.

Serious illnesses are often caused by a poor diet

No, eating a hamburger with a bottled juice is not a complete diet. Although the hamburger may contain vegetables, instead of a good diet it should be considered as an occasional treat. However, the problem comes when you eat this type of food frequently or, even worse, every day due to the lack of time to cook.

Many diseases are caused by condiments, improperly stored meats, an excess of sauces or sodas, among other foods or components that can be found in junk food sold on the streets. Colon cancer, diabetes, fatty liver, hepatitis and heart disease are just some of the serious diseases that can be contracted by eating fast food, both on the street and prepared at home. Since, if you eat meats, sausages and sodas (which are pre-processed foods) it is the same as you do it on the street or at home, because deep down you are eating incorrectly.

Thus, the main reason why there are a large number of people with hypertension and diabetes, among other diseases that are currently attacking humans, is a poor diet or, rather, a poor-quality diet.

Companies replace harmful additives with worse ones

You have probably seen the labels 'sugar free' or 'gluten free' on many foods. This, under normal conditions, would be positive for people who cannot ingest sugars, but there is a problem. And, according to Michael Polland, "companies replace saturated fat, excess sugar or gluten with artificial additives that are harmful to health." These substitutes are, in fact, more harmful than the natural components that they are substituting in the food in question.

For example, they can offer you a sugar-free soda with a chemical additive that simulates the taste of sugar, which is even worse than the sugar itself, which can also happen with fats that are replaced by a large amount of gluten. That is, it is a trick that many companies use to catch people like you, who want to take care of their diet. In the end they end up offering us a 'poisoned apple' that many of us have eaten out of innocence. The expert's recommendation in these cases is not to pay too much attention to the amount of calories, sugars or fats in each food, but to see them for what they are instead, foods that must be balanced to find harmony and a balanced diet.

It is difficult to find 100% healthy food

While it is rather difficult, it is not impossible to find a completely healthy diet, without artificial chemical additives or a high amount of sugars. You may be in a hurry when you leave for work and think of solving the day with a quick meal, but the solution to this is to prepare breakfast in advance. If possible, the night before, before going to bed, arrange a completely healthy meal. Of course, it is not advisable to eat preprocessed products on a regular basis, as they can be as harmful as fast food in some cases; food like fresh vegetables, meats with low percentages of fat and bought in reliable places, eggs and wholemeal flours are a better choice, among other products that have not gone through an industrial process of cooking or even injected with 'vitamins'.

Many believe that healthy foods have a higher cost, but it depends on how you look at it. If you want others to prepare healthy foods for you, yes, they will cost more than food for sale at a hot dog stand. But if you prepare them at home, with enough time and buying all the necessary ingredients yourself, then you will be feeding yourself properly at a low price. Nutrition specialist Maria Moreno, from the College of Dietitians of Navarra, says there is a very simple method to know if a preprocessed food is of good quality (though never excellent) or poor quality. The method consists of "looking at the label to know the additives; the longer the list, the poorer the quality of the product".

Problem foods behind the current obesity epidemic

A little more than a century ago, obesity was not a problem of global importance as it is today. While it was present in a number of regions, it was not present throughout the world. This is the case today and it is the result, in most cases, of the intake of foods high in sugars and fats. As mentioned above, even foods or beverages that claim to be sugar-free include sweeteners that can multiply their normal fat content, so you should not rely on them. However, in general terms, the main problem comes from a group of foods that are catalogued under the name of fast food, which are:

Corn puffs, among other packaged treats

The candies that are sold in packages are usually processed several times before they reach the commercial shelves. They go through various processes of cooking, frying and adding toppings to make their taste irresistible, but it is just this that alters the metabolism, as they are specifically created so that you do not get bored of eating them. Even if you have already eaten a considerable amount, you will continue to do so, thus blocking appetite control. It can be even worse if these treats come in the form of foods with large amounts of fat, salt, preservatives or sauces, such as a hot dog, pizza or hamburger (we categorize these types of foods as treats since the vitamins, proteins and minerals they can provide to the human body are very poor).

Fried food

Fried food, on the other hand, represents another problem of modern nutrition. According to a study held by the American Journal of Clinical Nutrition, an internationally popular health journal, "any diet that includes fried foods is predisposing the body to obesity". For this study, a sample of a little more than 40 thousand people was taken, reaching the conclusion that the consumption of this food group (fried foods) will negatively affect waist circumference and body mass index.

Fats, according to Gabriel Robledo, head of the research as a cardiologist, make the food tastier, something notorious if we compare frying with other healthier methods of food preparation, such as boiling or baking. On the other hand, fried foods generate a sensation of appetite, so they predispose you to keep eating even if you are no longer hungry. In addition, and this is where things get dangerous, fried foods make the body activate its nutrient absorption mechanism in an optimal way, with the consequence that they predispose it to absorb any other component that accompanies the fried food at the time of ingestion (salt or sauces, among other harmful elements in excess).

We are not saying that eating fried foods is a sin, but we do recommend not eating fried chips, chicken or cheese sticks (to give some examples) several times a week. The main preparation method for your food should be baking, steaming or grilling.

Energy drinks, sodas and bottled 'natural' juices.

Would you eat up to five tablespoons of sugar in a row in the morning, afternoon and evening? "Of course not," you may be thinking, as that is damaging to your health. However, industrially processed energy drinks, sodas and fruit juices include six to ten large spoonsful of sugar per liter on a beverage, especially if they are energy drinks. Sugary drinks of any kind that have been industrially bottled to last a good amount of time usually include empty calories, that is, they do not contribute anything to the body. And not only that, but also, when they are burned, the process is very slow and favors their rapid conversion into fat, thus increasing weight. Children, whose risk of obesity is especially high, will be 60% predisposed to develop obesity if they consume soft drinks on a daily basis.

Biscuits and bread

Within this category we will also include cookies, donuts and products with high levels of sugars and carbohydrates that include flour. These products, if not eaten on a regular basis, should not cause any harm; the problem arises when they are eaten every day or several times a week, especially when in addition to sugar they contain elements such as caramel, chocolate and syrups, ingredients that add a large percentage of sugar (which can be transformed into glucose and then into fats). While it is very harmful for the body to eat one high-calorie unit such as a donut, eating several will represent a great risk of developing obesity and diabetes in the medium or long term.

Candies, cakes, desserts and jellies

Foods classified as desserts are massively consumed every day by a large part of the world's population, since nowadays it is normal to consume a dessert after every meal. The reality is that they are not so healthy when after each meal you must consume one to feel satisfied. One or two a day are enough to stay healthy, as long as they are consumed in small quantities.

Jelly beans, chocolates, cake portions and jellies are the most dangerous when consumed every day after each main course and are not recommended for children. In addition, although it is not necessary to consume dessert so often, if you crave something sweet after every meal you can always opt for healthy homemade desserts. It is possible for you to know each of their ingredients and their levels of fats and sugars.

What is the main problem with today's meals?

Today's meals have two problems. The first is that they need to be ready quickly to feed a large number of people who need to eat on the go to go from one place to another with a full stomach; that is, there is no real importance given to food and no quiet time after the meal for the body to properly process the food. And since food needs to be prepared quickly and one of the fastest cooking methods available is frying, this way of cooking and eating is repeated in almost all (if not all) fast food chains around the world. Some of these chains, in addition to ingredients with excess fat, use unhealthy products in order to keep the food in a consumable state for a longer time, although they do not actually have vitamins or proteins usable by the body.

The second problem is similar to the first, but is focused on foods that are sold in supermarkets and contain, like fast food, preservatives to keep them fresh until people buy them. Within this category are canned goods, cured meats, some cheeses and some meats such as ready-to-cook hamburger patties. There is no doubt that it is healthier to buy food at the supermarket, but as long as it is not pre-processed. Because, although these contribute to the food being ready faster, you will be consuming fewer nutrients than buying fresh chicken, beef or fish, or vegetables in their natural state. With a shopping list based on healthy and natural products, you will also be contributing to the preservation of the environment by discarding foods that come in trays, unshelled or already cut.

It will be, of course, a little more tedious to clean the meats, season and cook them, but it will be much healthier than buying them ready-made in a supermarket, where these same meats or vegetables are given a chemical bath to avoid their rapid decomposition. In the case of meats, an additional percentage of fat may even be added to them so that they last longer and thus sell less percentage of meat with the same benefit.

Canned foods are not exempted from all this. You already know that foods that come in this state have been through a process of extraction of a good part of their natural nutrients to preserve them for longer and, in exchange, they have been injected with vitamins and minerals of lower quality. The result, obviously, is that the protein value will be much lower than buying the same food (for example, tuna) in its natural state. In the end, if we think that saving time is important, we must remember that our health is even more important. There will always be time to cook! Reserve at least one hour in your day to prepare your food. Over time, you will see how you will feel more energized to face each day, since this extra energy comes from the natural nutrients in abundance from the home-cooked meals you are eating.

Now that you know the importance of choosing your food and taking care of your diet, we will move on to talk about intermittent fasting, the method of eating that will help you lose weight and bring your glycemic index, body mass and fat levels to stable values.

CHAPTER II

History of intermittent fasting

Fasting has been practiced by man on repeated occasions throughout the history of mankind, motivated as much by natural causes as by religious, cultural, currents of thought or, in more modern times, by health issues. There are several ancient writings that indicate that fasting helped man to restore the health of the body, so intermittent fasting is not at all something that has emerged in the last century, but rather an ancient custom that has been well established today underpinned by various manuals for healthy eating that follow a set of well-described rules.

In some ruins in Egypt, Greece and India, writings and hieroglyphs have been found indicating that fasting served people to prevent diseases and unfavorable health conditions, linking it to a full way of life. During prehistoric times, cavemen gathered berries and hunted prey to sustain themselves, but there were times when they could not find sufficient sources of food, so people entered a period of starvation or natural fasting. In this way, the body was burning localized and stored fats for these emergency cases, so at the same time and in a chained way, they were lowering their fat and glucose reserves. It did not matter, then, that one day (or even two or more) they did not find food, since the cavemen's organism was familiar to a rhythm of life in which the possibility of not finding daily sources of food was real. This, on the other hand, does not happen today, where the body demands up to five meals a day.

In more modern times, going back to ancient Greece, physicians were convinced that the cure for any disease could be found in nature. An example of this is that, when an animal was sick, it stopped eating and preferred to rest and sleep to try to regenerate its health, so these doctors recommended their patients to do the same. In Greece, a very interesting finding took place: the phenomenon of hyper-concentration in the fasting state. According to what the Greeks discovered, when you are in a fasting state, your concentration improves your performance considerably. Just the opposite happens when you eat until you are satiated, causing a state of sleepiness and lethargy. In this era, intermittent fasting was also practiced in various religions. As we indicated before, the Christian religion focuses on Jesus Christ, who fasted for forty days with the sole intention of strengthening his relationship and communication with God (something that is associated with a period of maximum concentration and devotion). In Islam, a very different religion from Christianity, faithful Muslim's practice Ramadan, which consists of fasting for a month from sunrise to sunset, and eating only once a day during this nighttime schedule. Muslims have no problem with fasting; in fact, they do not even feel the need to eat more than once a day during Ramadan, as their bodies have become accustomed to intermittent fasting.

Returning to Egypt and the medicinal applications of fasting, there is evidence that in ancient times Egyptian doctors used fasting as a remedy to cure syphilis. But the existence of fasting in ancient times is not purely medicinal or religious. The Persians, for example, in their warrior division, ate only once a day, except for any type of meat. In turn, the warriors of Sparta began their training since childhood and in the process are deprived of meals as a method of early training. In the same way, only in adulthood, in Rome, soldiers fasted one day a week.

During the Middle Ages, different doctors came to the conclusion that fasting was the ultimate therapy to cure different diseases or prevent them. And we are not talking about just any doctor, but about eminences widely recognized between the 16th and 18th centuries in the field of medicine. One such case was that of Paracelsus, a Swiss physician who is considered one of the eminences of Western medicine. Paracelsus prescribed fasting to his patients and even came to consider this practice as a substitute for the medical professionals themselves. Not for nothing did he describe fasting as "the best of physicians, since it acts directly from within". Another distinguished 17th century physician, Dr. Friedrich Hoffmann, was one of the greatest advocates of fasting for health reasons and even published an essay entitled How to Cure Serious Diseases by Moderation in Eating and Fasting. In this essay, you can find different methods to cure diseases of the organism, mind and spirit, making it one of the most complete texts that had fasting as a main topic in the past.

During the 19th and 20th centuries, fasting for health purposes was at its peak. Both professional physicians and wise naturalists in natural remedies recommended fasting to maintain good health. This was mainly the case in Germany, where physicians recommended fasting in different facets of life. Dr. Von Seeland, for example, never tired of saying that fasting was a healing therapy of the highest level, while Dr. Christian Gustav, in one of his works, went so far as to write that "fasting is the most effective means of curing any disease". It serves as an example, moreover (among many other opinions of prominent naturalists and physicians on fasting in Germany at this time), the point of view defended by Dr. Möller, who stressed that "fasting is the only natural evolutionary method by which, with a systemic purification, physiological normality can be regained". In other words, fasting improves the body's own capacity for self-healing, freeing it from elevated levels of certain substances.

Also, during the nineteenth century, although in Switzerland, Dr. Von Segesser investigated fasting in depth in a sanatorium, reaching essential studies that were later expanded by Claude Louis Berthollet, a chemist and physician of the same nationality as the illustrious Von Segesser. Finally, another German, Dr. Hellmut Lützner, published a compilation of his experiences treating diseases and various health problems with fasting and resting. Some of his publications were the works Rebirth through fasting or Fasting therapy and nutritional therapy, two key studies that defended the theory that fasting provides a purification of high levels of free radicals, fats and sugars, eliminates inorganic elements from environmental pollution and even improves the appearance of the skin.

CHAPTER III

Scientific Foundations of Intermittent Fasting

Having cleared the previous concepts, it is the time to gradually develop practical, scientific, theoretical and intermittent fasting foundations, beginning to know simple terms that are will be continuously treated throughout this e-book. One of the major fundamentals of intermittent fasting can be observed in nature, specifically in carnivorous animals that have forced their metabolism to adapt to fasting when there are no valid food sources available. The lipogenesis is given both in animals and humans, it is a process consisting in the accumulation of fat to be to subsequently used as fuel if the body needs it because there is no new food intake. Therefore, both in animals and in humans (as some of the historical precedents that we have named) being fasting improves concentration, the reflexes and even the brainpower. This, without a doubt, helps to carry out tasks more quickly and thus get food, after which the body enters the process of rest. Apart from this, you're about to see some very interesting concepts about intermittent fasting, fasting in general, food and health, which will help you understand each type of intermittent fasting and how they are carried out.

What is hunger?

Sometimes you feel your stomach gradually start to burn until it reaches a point where it begins to ' grunt ' for food. This happens when there is hunger, a natural alarm that indicates that the body needs food to replenish the energy it has lost throughout the day. Now, hunger can appear at different times of the day and the most logical action would be to calm it. For this reason, many people eat up to six times a day, three main meals and three light meals. This is done in order not to avoid hunger, but to ' accelerate the metabolism ', as they say. However, this last statement is a fallacy and we will explain why.

Is eating 6 times a day discouraged?

At the time of eating, insulin is produced, which is a substance that helps the body to capture all the proteins and vitamins from food, taking them to the cells responsible for their absorption. If during the day you eat abundantly or, worse, so very often and in large quantities, the cells of the body will warn the body that it no longer needs energy because it is sufficiently acquired. If after this, the insulin continues to transport nutrients, both the cells and the liver will warn that they should take them away for storage to so use them when there is no energy available, either from lack of food or strenuous activities that require one lot of energy.

The energy transported is immediately transformed into fat, which is commonly located in areas such as the abdomen, buttocks, the thighs and the legs, with the result that we all are familiar with: a fattening individual. The solution to this problem is simple; to not to get fat, we must simply limit the amount of food that we carry to our cells. That way, we began to consume enough to keep us active and healthy, and only when stocks are running low will have to eat again to replenish the energy used. So, if you already are in an obesity profile, you should not worry, as intermittent fasting can help you use these fat reserves that you have accumulated and your body will gradually get used to the fact that it is not necessary to eat six times a day.

What do we recommend then? We simply recommend people to make three main meals with excellent protein content, with good fats and carbohydrates. And if you are a slugabed, try to have lunch from 12 to 13, for example, and to dinner between 18 and 19 hours.

Is hunger really a mental problem?

The quick answer to this question is 'no'. Whoever is hungry is perfectly sane in their mind, they just need to get used the new patterns of foods that are about to become a very healthy lifestyle. Normally it is believed, that when feeling that itching in the stomach, it is necessary to eat since it is a warning that our body sends us that there is a lack of energy. In fact, it is inevitable to feel that sensation throughout the day. We imagine the stomach as a gasoline tank of a vehicle: the more it is filled with fuel; the needle gets closer to the region that indicates that the tank is completely full. Now well, when hunger appears we normally think we are about to faint, as the ' vehicle ' which is our body has been virtually with no energy or 'with the needle at zero', so it is to add necessary food in it so it can keep working. All of this makes sense for those who do not know how the human body works, but the fact is that, unlike a car, the human body has significant reserves of energy so that, if there is no food, it can keep running for a few more days.

There are studies that have found that it may be a good idea to fast during the morning, because during these hours hunger can be easily controlled, unlike the last hours of the afternoon or beginning of the evening. Afternoon and evening, as manifested by people who have started a diet regimen, are more difficult to control food cravings or hunger itself. This happens even if in the previous night they have not eaten anything and neither in the morning. That is why you should know that when wanting to skip dinner, you will feel a greater sense of hunger. We can ensure, therefore, that hunger is not an automatic indicator of the moment when the body has run out of energy (it does not work like a car), but an involuntary reflex learned over generations and generations. This can be easily explained. Just think of a grilled steak that gives off an exquisite smoky aroma and whose drops that fall on the coals make the aroma even more attractive. I am sure that imagining this, even if you ate about three hours ago, you will get a huge appetite, even if right now your body is still processing the nutrients from the last meal.

This phenomenon is not something new and, in fact, it was studied several decades ago, specifically in the 1980s, by the scientist Ivan Palov. In this study, Pavlov analyzed salivation of dogs in natural conditions and their salivation when lunchtime approached, when they saw that someone was preparing a meal or when they put the plate full of food in front of them. The studies yielded conclusive results: salivation increased as they viewed food. Something like this happens to us when we see something that we find delicious. Although we are not hungry our mind begins to imagine the taste of the dish and thus ends up causing the feeling of hunger. And this explains, ultimately, that hunger is not related to the gross energy levels of the body.

But hunger is not really the only sensation that appears when seeing food, hearing the sounds related to eating or smelling its aroma. Other phenomena in the body also happen, such as increased pancreatic secretion, insulin production and, of course, excessive salivation, which is not but a symptom that the body is preparing to receive food and process it in the form of food bolus (for which a good amount of enzymes from saliva is necessary). Have you ever wondered why do shops that sell food present it in an attractive way? Yes, maybe a nice presentation sells more, but there is another reason, and it is that the mere fact of seeing the food presented in an elegant way produces a greater sense of hunger and, therefore, a greater sense of relief when eating, which will gradually make the client return to the business premises to repeat the experience Even in many restaurants it has become fashionable to prepare your own dish, where people can select the ingredients they want for their meal. This is a great way to do business since people often take in food more through their eyes than through their stomachs. As a result, we fill our plate to the brim with the food that looks and smells the most appetizing.

This is also seen in animals. Specifically, in Palov's study it was determined that just by seeing an empty dish in its owner's hand a dog could begin to feel anxiety and extra salivation. This sensation, not surprisingly, increased as the time when food was normally provided during the day approached, as the dog knew it was time to get fed. The same thing happens to us humans. As 8:00 a.m., 12:00 noon or 6:00 p.m. approaches (schedules may vary according to cultures and the rhythm of life of each one, although they are some of the most widespread) the body lets us know through hunger that it is already the time when it usually receives food, so it demands it through the sensation of hunger without caring much if it has been eaten a few hours ago.

Now, we must ask ourselves one question: Is hunger truly real? This is how the time comes to debunk the myth, since this type of hunger is nothing more than a behavior learned by the organism based on months, years or decades of following the same pattern. This behavior is especially marked if in your environment you have food within easy, fast or continuous reach (such as junk food or when you find yourself watching someone else prepare a dish assiduously). For real hunger to make its appearance, the body must enter a state of starvation, a state that only arises when most of the body's energy reserves disappear, giving way to the consumption of nutrients that should not be consumed. And this only occurs after more than 24 hours without food.

Have you ever noticed how children prefer not to eat in the mornings because they simply have no appetite? Their little bodies have not yet been used to the morning feeding regimen so the body does not demand the food typical of this schedule! Another characteristic of 'mental hunger', as we might call it, is that it usually does not appear when we are carrying out activities that require a high level of concentration or physical demand, but appears just after these activities are finished. The reason? The mind was engaged in a more important activity than following a previously learned pattern of behavior, so it directed its energies to this activity (as does the brain in a fasting state).

Of course, it is not in the best interest of the big fast-food chains to keep people on an intermittent fasting regime, so they invite them to eat morning, noon and night those dishes that they themselves have created especially for each schedule. In order to sell their products (food), they will use any method they have at their disposal, from promoting their food with free samples to advertisements in which we see how someone eats or disclosing how the food is prepared, among other signals that the brain quickly interprets as an invitation to eat or as an approximation of the meal schedule. Now, even knowing as you do that you are actually fighting a natural body response to an eating behavior you've been engaging in for decades, you may be wondering: How do you fight these signals from your mind?

Nipping 'mental hunger' in the bud

An unhealthy habit is broken by challenging it with a habit that is healthy, even if the process of adaptation is somewhat hard. It is not necessary to skip breakfast every day; you can skip breakfast one day, lunch the next day and dinner the following day, all in order to eliminate the food habit from our body and reactivate the body's capacity to feed itself in the absence of food (as in ancient times). By eliminating the food habit from the body, hunger will appear only at times when we are really hungry and not out of habit. This is achieved after a few months practicing intermittent fasting, which does not have to be understood as a different regime of eating schedules, but as a process by which you skip one or two meals a day to lose weight, accustom the body to use energy reserves and learn to distinguish real hunger from that resulting from various stimuli.

We also leave you a trick that will help you avoid the feeling of hunger that is born when you feel this stimulation: eat only when you are sitting at the table. This will help prevent you from snacking while watching a game on the couch, in bed while watching a movie or on the street when you smell the aroma of a freshly baked pizza. Stop falling prey to external stimulation! Get your mind in the habit starting today that food is reserved for the table only, so that hunger will appear when your body actually needs food and sitting down at the table will further open up your appetite (and not in other places that encourage junk food consumption).

In any case, it is advisable not to take too hard the creation of a new habit, whatever it is, as this requires some time. Do not pretend to eliminate the habit of eating every day at nine o'clock at night if you have been doing it for eight years! It is advisable to take it one step at a time. Start by lowering the amount of food you eat during a certain time of the day and a week later start to eliminate completely that meal of the day (which should not be only the one of a specific time). At the beginning, the 'mental hunger' will appear, since the body misses the food that was supplied at the usual time of day, but little by little you will see that this sensation will disappear. In addition, you should not worry about excessive self-demand, because you can eat or drink any of the ingredients that we recommend to make this feeling disappear until the next meal.

Can hunger be avoided while my body gets used to fasting?

Instead of snacking or munching between meals, try eating main meals that keep you satiated for longer, so that hunger comes just when it's time to eat another main course. One of the most important components to ensure that you stay full longer is fat, although it may seem counterproductive. With fat, your stomach and insulin will be kept busy processing it, whereas it will be used up quickly if you stay active throughout the day (exercising, on the way to work, working, and so on). Some food and ingredients that contain fat by nature and that can be added to your daily diet are:

- White or yellow cheeses (especially of the mozzarella variety).
- Butter.
- Olives.
- Seeds and nuts.
- Sources of healthy natural oils, such as olive oil.
- Mayonnaise.

In addition to fat, there are other ingredients that you can add to the three main dishes each day. Some of them may be the following:

- **Quinoa:** quinoa is an ingredient that you will surely have heard of before if you have already done some dieting, which is not strange at all since it is extremely tasty when mixed with other ingredients. It contains no sugars and has a good amount of protein and fiber. In addition, its carbohydrates are complex and very usable by the body, so its digestion requires more time and you will last longer satisfied.
- **Lentils:** lentils are very appreciated in a great variety of diets since, in addition to being very tasty they can be prepared in a great number of ways, from soups to emulating the shape and flavor of grilled hamburger meat. 100 grams of lentils can provide your body with about 8 grams of fiber and 9 grams of protein. Of course, they will take time to digest, so you will stay fuller longer, although it is not advisable to eat them when you are going to carry out strenuous activities afterwards, such as exercise, climbing or long walks.
- **Hummus:** hummus is a perfect additive that can be the ideal substitute for traditional sauces. It is rich in fiber, which allows you to stay satiated for several hours, in addition to providing the body with a good amount of protein and healthy fats. You need to try it!
- **Avocado**: avocado has a light, creamy and somewhat fatty fla-

vor that can be ideal in the company of other foods, but the truth is that its benefits do not end there. What if we told you that it also has about 5 grams of protein per 300 grams, and a good amount of potassium, so it helps improve nerve response and muscle contraction? What are you waiting to add it to your meals?

- **Barley**: Barley is a type of grain that will make you feel full for several hours if you include a good amount in your meals. It is also rich in protein and fiber and can be mixed with different drinks or dishes.

Water as an ally in fasting

Sometimes we may confuse thirst with the desire to eat. This will logically cause us to eat food out of schedule, thus increasing the amount of fats and sugars that will promote obesity. It is convenient, therefore, that before eating you drink a glass of water so you can make sure if you are really hungry or just thirsty. Another powerful way to use water to avoid breaking the fast is to drink a glass of water one or two hours after the meal. This will soften hunger. You can also drink other types of beverages, such as black coffee, tea and flavored water. By drinking water and engaging in other activities you may find that the hunger will go away in a few minutes, but if it doesn't, there is a trick that rarely fails: drink a spoonful of apple cider vinegar and lemon.

You may be skeptical at first, but the truth is that by drinking just one tablespoon of apple cider vinegar your hunger will disappear in the space of an hour without you having to do anything else. Moreover, preparing this miraculous spoonful to avoid hunger is simple: just mix some apple cider vinegar with water and drink a spoonful as a remedy. The apple cider vinegar will act as an insulator between the gastric acids and the walls of the stomach, thus preventing ulcers in the first periods of fasting, while the body gets used to the new diet. To increase the effect of this remedy, in the same glass where you mixed the apple cider vinegar and water, add about four drops of lemon juice and mix well. You will see how this beverage will help you achieve your goal of eating only three meals a day when it seemed impossible to do so.

What are electrolytes and how can they help me reduce my hunger?

If we talk about avoiding feeling hungry, it is possible not to talk about electrolytes, as they are nutrients that the body needs for everything to go well in the day to day. Proteins are not the only nutrient that will activate and regenerate the body after a tedious day's work, because electrolytes do that too. Some well-known electrolytes are magnesium, calcium and potassium, and the human body is especially sensitive to the levels of all of them; if one is missing, the alarm called hunger will immediately begin to sound (and make itself felt) in the body. When your body is lacking these electrolytes, it will be normal to feel the need for sweet foods or foods with large amounts of saturated fats, which are just the typical cravings for sweets or fast food.

Some drinks can replenish the electrolytes you have lost during the day and thus prolong a state of satiated appetite. Some of the most popular drinks for this purpose are Powerade, Aquarius or Gatorade, and there are even powdered electrolyte packets with a delicious fruit flavor and no added sugars.

The solution to alleviate hunger at the beginning of intermittent fasting

It is often difficult to control periods of hunger at the beginning of intermittent fasting. It may even take two to four months to get used to it completely, but after this adaptation phase your body will have become accustomed to using all the available energy supplied by food without the need to make unnecessary reserves of nutrients in the form of fat.

Emotional hunger and how to identify it

The so-called emotional hunger is more linked to feelings or moods than to an established habit. This type of hunger appears when one feels happy, sad, tired, angry or anxious, among other moods that can be experienced throughout the day. Therefore, it can be conceptualized as the act of eating in order to find a sense of relief, even if one does not eat a single meal or is not hungry. This emotional hunger can appear throughout the day as a result of simple boredom, stress, doing monotonous or repetitive things or due to strong emotions. And food, in these cases, seeks to make a pause to a fun activity or comfort through a snack, although there is also the well-known thought of "I deserve it since this is what I work for". These feelings usually end up generating discomfort in the person who ends up succumbing to the temptation to take a snack unhealthy for their health, either by having spent unnecessary money on it, by breaking the diet or both situations.

The worst thing is that when you eat because of emotional hunger you may finish a dish, but after an hour or two you may feel hungry again. This happens because hunger does not come from the need for food, but from the need for a reward, a break or comfort for the current mood. You can self-examine by asking yourself the following questions:

- Do I usually snack when I am bored?
- In times of stress do I usually eat something to de-stress?
- Do you celebrate your accomplishments, no matter how small, by having a snack?

Differences between real hunger, mental hunger and emotional hunger

Humans have three different types of hunger, each of which can strike throughout the day, although real hunger may not strike unless you are struggling financially, on a demanding diet, or practicing intermittent fasting for periods of more than sixteen hours. Below, we will discuss the characteristics of these three types of hunger. Namely:

Emotional hunger

Emotional hunger is born, as its name suggests, from emotions that can occur throughout the day. It usually appears when you suffer from boredom, stress, anxiety or sadness, but it can occur perfectly well in other moments that generate some kind of emotion. This type of hunger appears suddenly, since it is associated to an emotional stimulus. It is also typical of emotional hunger the fact that you are not hungry for real, healthy, homemade or natural food, but for pizza, sushi or hamburgers, among other specific foods.

Mental hunger or for habit

This type of hunger goes hand in hand with our body's biological clock. When the time has come in which we commonly take food to our mouth and at a given moment it is not happening, the well-known sensation of hunger begins, which does not increase, but remains there as if it were part of a whim of the organism. This type of hunger also appears due to external stimuli such as those mentioned above if mealtime is near.

Real hunger

Real hunger is the one that appears when several hours have passed without providing food to the body and it has already exhausted most of the glucose (fat) deposits in it. Real hunger can appear after twenty-four hours of fasting, sometimes more and sometimes less, because it depends on the amount of energy that the person who practices fasting has accumulated in the body. This type of hunger, the real hunger, is very rarely felt in a cycle of constant eating by a person with a careless diet, but when it comes it is better to follow the warning and consume food in order to avoid muscle loss and that the body feeds on localized fat in regions where you do not want to lose volume. Remember that the body is very intelligent and, in the absence of food, it will look for sources of energy anywhere, even if it ends up weighing on the body's general health and, in extreme cases, on life.

Will I be hungry when I start fasting?

We're not going to lie to you: you will feel hungry during the first and even the second or third week after you start intermittent fasting. Although it can be mitigated, there will always be either emotional hunger or mental hunger, the product of a lifestyle with uncontrolled eating cycles for so long. But, despite this, the truth is that it is not a terrible and unbearable process, but quite bearable. If you think that the hunger that starts as a craving will increase so much that you will feel as if your stomach is being pierced, we deny this, since you will not experience this type of hunger, which is the real one, but a hunger product of a craving for fries, hamburgers or simply for eating at times that are no longer approved.

The key to control false hunger is to identify it immediately and discover the lie often self-imposed with sentences or thoughts such as: "It is for my health; I must eat or I will faint/lose muscle/lower my defenses". When you feel any kind of hunger you should ask yourself the following questions:

- Is it appropriate for me to eat at this time?
- Did I see something appealing and want to try it, even if it is outside my mealtime?
- Do I feel bored, sad or anxious and need to eat to compensate for the feeling?

By asking yourself these questions you will effectively unmask false hunger, remembering that not every time you get hungry it has to be false hunger. It may be that your body has exhausted its energy reserves after an activity that required a great effort, so always ask yourself before eating and remember that sometimes it is only necessary to drink some tea, coffee or natural juice without sugar to calm this feeling of hunger.

The good news is that after about three weeks of fasting your body will begin to get used to this new diet, thus disappearing the emotional or habit hunger and leaving only the real hunger, which you will not have to feel if you know that with a glass of tea or natural juice it can disappear.

What happens to our body when we fast?

"You may faint", "You will spend the whole day with low energy" and/or "You will start to lose muscle" are some of the lies that are usually heard when talking about fasting. However, the process of autophagy is something totally natural as the human body manages to adapt to a new metabolic process. The benefits of intermittent fasting can be seen after a constant fasting period of 12 hours and longer, which can extend up to two days without food. Next, we will see what happens in the organism when it begins to get used to each of these time varieties.

What happens to the body if you fast for 12 hours?

The daily fast of 10 to 12 hours will be the first step to transform fats into energy. After this period of time, the fat begins, little by little, to turn into energy, which passes directly into the bloodstream feeding the rest of the organs as if you had just eaten. If we also consider that fat is also burned while sleeping, then this fasting can be perfectly coupled to the time of sleep, during which we will rarely feel hungry. An example of a fast of this interval can be fasting from 9 pm at night until 9 am the next day, so that you only get to experience hunger for an hour or two at the beginning of the practice of intermittent fasting (which you can mitigate with the tricks that we recommend). However, after a few months or even weeks you will no longer feel hungry until 9 o'clock in the morning as your body will be completely used to this new eating schedule/habit.

What happens to the body after an ideal 16-hour fast?

Fasting for 16 hours is the standard intermittent fasting for each day. By fasting for this time interval you will achieve great benefits in terms of weight loss and energy utilization, although, we do not recommend fasting from the start in this way, as the body will not be used to it and the periods of hunger will be very intense.

This 16-hour interval is normally for men, while women fast up to 14 hours a day, at least within the Leagains diet model. In any case, this intermittent fasting will burn large amounts of calories during the night and morning, since after dinner (which may be at 8 pm) nothing will be eaten again until lunch the next day. In addition, with this type of diet you will not only burn fat, but you will also avoid recurrent obesity (if you are coming off one), you will be able to stay at your ideal weight and the levels of fat and sugar in the body will be normalized. Not to mention that you will be preventing liver disease and heart abnormalities.

Fasting for several days and its advantages

People who decide to fast strongly for a maximum of two days a week will be able to see the benefits of intermittent fasting quickly, as this type of diet burns a large amount of fat in a short time. However, pay close attention, as all fasting intervals must be monitored and controlled to avoid nutritional problems. In this interval are found, for example, people who execute an intermittent fasting of 12 or 16 hours for two days a week depriving themselves of foods rich in carbohydrates or fats and consuming just 600 grams of calories per day. In other words, during these intense fasting days you eat, but significantly reduce the amount of calories you normally consume.

The fasting effects of this diet -also known as fast diet- are several: the drastic reduction in insulin levels, insulin sensitivity and, of course, an accelerated weight reduction. The interesting thing about this diet is that, according to the results of a study involving 107 women who practiced it, eating few calories for two days had the same effects as a more rigorous diet, such as restricting calories every day of the week. In other words, intensity has an effect.

What happens in the body with an interdaily fast?

Interday fasting for some people is the main face of intermittent fasting, as it is given alternately every two days, with the person choosing whether to consume food during that day up to 500 calories or, on the contrary, avoid any type of food and barely ingest water or electrolyte-based beverages. Of course, during the two days that the person decides not to fast, they can eat their three main dishes a day with as much healthy food as they wish, respecting the fasting day when appropriate as part of the lifestyle.

With this fasting it is possible to maintain an ideal weight, lose weight in a sustained manner until reaching an ideal weight and prevent heart disease or keep the body healthy to avoid heart attacks, if you already suffer from a heart disease or there are risks. Some nutritionists had their doubts about the effectiveness of this type of fasting, but with time and based on studies they discovered that, in a group of 32 people, there was an average weight loss of 5 kilograms after only three months, which proved its effectiveness. However, giving up a single day to eat 500 calories or even no solid food at all can be very demanding for someone who is just starting to fast, so you will need to gain previous experience with less demanding fasts first.

Apart from these intermittent fasts in different time ranges, there are other fasts that offer more or less the same benefits to the body when practiced, but they will be addressed later, when talking about the types of intermittent fasts, how to practice them and how to feed yourself while practicing them. As a summary of the biological processes that the human body undergoes when subjected to this fasting we can say that autophagy takes place, the process by which the body depletes its own energy reserves (localized fat in different areas). This occurs to the point that the body fat index reaches its healthy levels and the energy of the three main meals is fully utilized without being saved, for the simple reason that no more food than necessary is ingested.

All the benefits and advantages of fasting

Although we have already addressed some of the processes that happen in the body, as soon as you start fasting under the intermittent fasting regimen, you have not yet deepened in the general benefits of fasting, those that are linked to the lifestyle of the person who has adopted fasting in a definitive way. Since the benefits are diverse, we have organized them into several points.

Fasting helps end emotional hunger

If you are hungry because of something you have experienced, such as anxiety, sadness or happiness, then you may be suffering from emotional hunger, an eating disorder linked to the process of dealing with different types of everyday situations on a daily basis. It may be that feeling shut down, bored, or downhearted pushes you to eat to 'fill' that emotional void, which in turn triggers a fat storage response in the body on a recurring basis depending on the periodicity with which this extra eating occurs. But this emotional hunger is also linked to uncontrolled eating schedules, since people with this disorder eat a snack several times a day and it seems totally normal to them.

With a programmed fast you can control the episodes of emotional hunger and avoid eating any type of food during the period of time in question, so you will respect more this previously programmed time. Once you are over the stage where you have to discipline your body to understand that meals are only taken at certain times, you will no longer have to make any additional effort. Your body will let you know when it needs food and the best thing is that it will only be at the three hours of the day when a main meal is due.

Intermittent fasting increases and improves immune system functions

The continuous consumption of fast food, among other unhealthy foods for the body, causes free radicals to multiply at an accelerated rate. Free radicals are a set of molecules resulting from the body's daily cellular processes. Although the molecules allow cellular and molecular processes to occur correctly, over time these free radicals gather as a result of cellular respiration, affecting the membranes of normal cells, altering their molecular structure and triggering adverse effects in the body.

Fortunately, the process of intermittent fasting not only slows down the production of free radicals, but months after implementing this lifestyle it will be possible for the levels of radicals to be dramatically reduced. This happens because fewer and fewer of these molecules gather and those that are already affecting the molecular structure of the cells are processed and disappear. In fact, in the animal world it is possible to observe, for example, that when a dog feels some kind of discomfort or pain it prefers to rest and stop eating, since by instinct it knows that its organism will stabilize the substances, deficiencies or excesses that make it feel sick. Therefore, if fasting is part of your daily routine, you will be protected against diseases and, in case one appears, your body will be able to attack it from the very first moment thanks to the fasting periods.

Do you think that not stopping eating for a period of time while you are sick is counterproductive? The truth is that it depends on the situation. If you stop eating, say, fast food, fatty and canned foods, and replace them with other foods that will give your body the nutrition it needs, you will end up seeing a significant improvement in your state of health even if you only eat two meals a day. And this will also be beneficial for your body's defenses, as long as you combine good nutrition and fasting with proper rest periods, of course.

Controlled fasting will help you lose weight and keep it off

Perhaps this is the benefit you were waiting to read about, since it is one of the greatest desires of people interested in fasting. Intermittent fasting will help you lose those extra pounds that are affecting your figure and even help you stay at your ideal weight without having to suffer from hunger or eating food that you do not like as with traditional diets. However, you will feel hungry during the first months, during the period in which your body will get used to a new diet, something fully controllable by ingesting fiber and calories in a responsible amount, which will help you feel fuller for longer.

It may seem miraculous, but it is proven that depriving yourself of a meal or two, eating only 500 grams of food a day or doing a complete fast based on electrolyte-rich drinks can quickly attack the fat deposits located in all areas of your body, thus achieving a uniform weight reduction. You already know the explanation why this happens: the body uses stored energy in the absence of a direct food source, such as any of the traditional three meals a day. By not ingesting food between the main meals - for example, between lunch and dinner - the body uses fat reserves, burning them and injecting these nutrients into the blood. In short, your body's main fuel will switch from glucose to reserved fats during the first few months of fasting in any of its modes. Once you have reached a low body fat index, your body will take energy directly from meals (from the sugar, fats, carbohydrates and vitamins contained in each dish). During this last period, you can relax intermittent fasting, although it should never be abandoned if you want to maintain your ideal weight.

Intermittent fasting will lower your blood sugar levels

As if that were not enough, if you have high blood sugar levels, with intermittent fasting you will be able to lower and control them thanks to its effectiveness in improving insulin sensitivity. By programmed fasting, insulin is able to optimally process carbohydrates and give orders to the cells to feed the body with the glucose that travels through the bloodstream. Thanks to this, and after a medical consultation, you will be able to avoid major problems such as diabetes or future predisposition to it.

Fasting will give your stomach and digestive system in general a rest.

The digestive system is made up of very complex parts that should be allowed to rest from time to time. In fact, by giving your digestive system a rest period, it can better prepare itself to digest food and waste from the digestion process. However, if your stomach is constantly working on digesting sweets, desserts, snacks and main meals, then the digestion process may not be 100% effective resulting in the fats from these foods not being fully digested and going straight to storage. In other words, contrary to popular belief, constant eating only prevents the digestive system from taking breaks, which will affect its functioning and fat processing capacity. In addition, it will negatively affect your metabolism. This is why intermittent fasting will optimize all of your body's digestive processes.

Does it help you live longer?

It may seem contradictory, but fasting will help you live longer. Scientists at Harvard University, in the United States, have discovered that practically "the more you eat the less time you have to live". How did they reach this conclusion? By analyzing the life expectancy of various communities around the world and contrasting it with their respective diets. They also determined that the more food you eat during your youth, the more your digestive system will be affected and, therefore, your metabolism will be slowed down. Of course, people who eat healthy without intermittent fasting will also be affected due to this aging of the digestive system, although in a less harmful way than those who are used to eating fast food on a regular basis.

But among all these groups, the most benefited is undoubtedly the one that performs intermittent fasting, since with intermittent fasting you will not only be eating healthily, but you will be allowing your digestive system to rest to process new carbohydrates and proteins in an optimal way, thus avoiding gaining weight due to not processing fats resulting from eating all day long.

It is a depurative method

We have already mentioned it above, but we cannot fail to remember the fact that one of the most powerful advantages of fasting is the depuration of our own organism and without the need of drugs or external ingredients. Our body will be in charge of consuming all the remains of fat and free radicals in order to obtain the necessary energy to be able to function. If you wish, you can call this process 'activating the survival mode', although it may sound a bit extreme.

At first, we know that it will be hard to feel real hunger (yes, real because what you usually feel between meals is nothing but food cravings), but by consuming dishes rich in fiber and hard-to-digest carbohydrates you can stay full until your body gets used to the right eating hours. These times are breakfast, lunch and dinner or directly lunch and dinner if you practice demanding intermittent fasting and fully focused on the elimination of fats. Scientific studies sustain that for a person to feel hungry, 12 to 24 hours of starvation are necessary; therefore, if you feel 'hungry' before, it is nothing but a reflection of the body to the routine to which you have accustomed it, which is precisely eating every few hours.

Improve concentration for practicing various spiritual or functional activities

Some people claim that by fasting they can increase their concentration abilities to perform various activities; in addition, the spiritual connection related to the beliefs of each person can be encouraged. Sportsmen who practice hiking or natural exploration or people who are fond of meditation, yoga or martial arts have intermittent fasting as a daily practice, since it helps them to focus on their activities in an optimal way. The reason for this was investigated for a long time by scientists until they found the answer, which is as simple as the amount of energy consumed by the digestion process takes a good part of the body's energy. This is the explanation why fasting improves concentration or functional capacities, as it provides the body with significant energy savings. The energies saved from the digestive process can be used for other activities, as long as the person eats healthily within the recommended time range for intermittent fasting.

Improves the appearance of the skin

There is no better treatment to improve skin health than regular fasting. Toxins normally deposit in the skin as a result of environmental pollution, which age the complexion and make the skin dry. Interestingly, fasting completely for 24 hours has yielded surprising results in people with dry skin. This happens because the energy that would normally be channeled to the digestive system is channeled to other parts of the body, one of them being the skin (which becomes freer of these toxins).

But actually not only the skin is positively affected by fasting; there is also a positive impact of fasting on organs such as the liver and kidneys, which need to rest from their daily work, especially if you eat unhealthy food and drink sodas or processed juices.

It saves you a good part of your income

Have you ever sat down with a notebook and pencil and calculated how much you spend on fast food every month? If you had, you would be certainly surprised by the amount of money that comes out of your pocket on this type of unhealthy food, money that you could have spent buying natural ingredients with active nutrients. We invite you, therefore, to carry out a very interesting activity: calculate the amount of money you currently spend on fast food (if you are a regular consumer of this type of food) and allocate the same budget on ingredients to prepare homemade food. Over time, you will see how the money not only pays off, but you will have more energy and lose weight with the help of intermittent fasting.

Other benefits of intermittent fasting you need to know

Although the benefits of intermittent fasting that have been listed may seem quite a few (these are some of the most notable), the truth is that there are even more. The list does not end here. Other benefits of this healthy lifestyle that intermittent fasting brings are the following:

- It greatly reduces bad cholesterol.
- It reduces localized swelling in certain areas of the body.
- Reduces the possibility of neuron death.
- It reduces the possibility of the appearance or multiplication of cells related to cancer.
- It improves the capacity of self-control before certain impulses promoting discipline.

CHAPTER IV

The relationship between metabolism and fasting

One of the most important and least known topics when it comes to focusing on our nutritional health is the relationship between fasting and metabolism. Typically, people believe that the more they eat, the faster their metabolism becomes; as the digestive system has to process a large amount of food continuously, forcing it to work quickly. However, this theory is incorrect. When a person does not let his digestive system rest, it is not that it works in an accelerated way, increasing metabolism, but that it processes nutrients and food in general in an ineffective way. In the long run it makes the metabolism slower and slower, as the digestive system is constantly used and it ages.

Contrary to popular belief, when a people cannot get food, their bodies goes into the so - called ' mode of survival ' , under which the body adapts to the new reality and take advantage of any reserves of energy possible to cope with this period of starvation. During the fasting process there are three main proteins that interact to improve metabolism. One of them is known as the stress hormone cortisol, another is responsible for detecting fatty acids so that they can be used by the body and, finally, there is a third one that detects cellular energy. This last protein has been baptized as AMPK, and has the important task of scanning the body to find other proteins and sources of reusable energy when there is no food. Its structure is especially complex and has been found to be essential for providing energy to the body during fasting.

As to be fasting as a lifestyle, these three distinctive proteins are getting stronger and are optimizing their search processes of energy sources. Eventually, these proteins will find in the liver the main source of energy in the fasting state, which through the process of gluconeogenesis take stored sugars to transform them into energy. According to various studies, in the body of one individual of about

70 kilos (154 pounds) weight and 1.70 meters (5,5") high, there are 300g (2.4 oz) of glucide (which last one day), 11 kilos (24 pounds) of lipid (lasting up to 40 days) and 10 kilos (22 pounds) of proteins that are practically stable in the body. That happens, under normal circumstances, only when you are not fasting. Now, you may be wondering what happens when you start fasting. Simply, the body is fed especially from lipids, employs the energy reserves without retaining additional water of the food and seals all possible leaks of vitamins, holding them for 'emergency cases'.

Metabolic phases of fasting

During fasting, three basic metabolic phases can be experienced. In the first phase, the human body is fueled by glucose and other carbohydrates. This glucose circulating in the body, given by the recently consumed food, is gradually used up until there is none left. After this, the reserves of the liver are consumed, which can take up to two days to be completely consumed. If in two days a person does not eat, then he or she will go into hypoglycaemia (the well-known sugar crash). You will know that you really need to eat when the classic symptoms of low blood sugar appear, mainly cold sweats and dizziness. During this first phase, however, localized fats in the body are not usually consumed.

During the second metabolic phase of fasting, the body begins to feed on lipids because the body has entered the so-called hypoglycemia, the lack of nutrients from foods that should be entering the body and are not doing so. In this phase, the hypothalamus acts by releasing certain hormones, such as growth hormone and stimulating lipolytic and ketogenic actions, which prevent proteins from being metabolized. The adrenal glands are also stimulated, which produce an increase in catecholamines. This, in turn, promotes glycogenesis (the name given to the processing of reserved energy) especially in the muscles and liver, while decreasing insulin secretion. During this second phase, an increase in glucocorticoid functions is also produced, generating absorption of amino acids from the liver and the release of amino acids coming from proteins. Finally, the pancreas responds; specifically, it decreases insulin and increases glucagon, which is a hormone that serves to regulate blood glucose.

The third phase is a stage in which it is necessary to eat, otherwise the body will fall into a state of starvation, the unhealthy point in any fast. In this third stage, the human organism will have made every effort to burn all the energy reserves at its disposal, until there are practically none left. This is why edema may appear at this limit stage, if the fast has been forced into prolonged starvation. In summary, it is possible to identify the phases of fasting in a simple way by following these points:

- **First phase.** During this phase the food is consumed. About 1200 calories normally last 24 hours, so the body will be able to withstand a day without eating with a diet based on this number of calories. And, since it is proportional to the diet followed, if 2000 calories are consumed your body could last up to 40 or 48 hours.
- **Second phase.** This is the phase in which the body begins to enter fasting and starts to stimulate the metabolic function of organs such as the pancreas, the nerves, the adrenal glands and the hypothalamus. All this in order to consume lipids and fatty acids. Proteins are affected during the first hours of fasting, however after a prolonged period of fasting the consumption of proteins by the body is minimal.
- **Third phase.** During the third phase, the body enters a state of starvation. In an attempt to survive, the organism begins to feed on proteins that are necessary for other processes, such as the repair of muscle tissue. This is why there is a significant loss of muscle mass and the subsequent death of the individual if the fasting is not brought to an end as soon as possible. This phase can be called the border phase, since it marks the end of a fasting cycle and the beginning of a new fasting process after ingesting the food required by the organism to survive.

How long can the body tolerate fasting metabolically speaking?

A lot of people believe that by fasting they will quickly go into a context of vitamin deficiency, but this has been proven to be false, since no person who has fasted has died due to lack of vitamins. Studies also show that the human body can tolerate between 40 and 60 days under prolonged and intermittent fasting, although there are cases where obese people have gone up to a year under severe intermittent fasting.

Fasting and lost electrolytes

It has been proven that during fasting up to 10% of the body's water can be lost considering the individual's weight, which would cause a significant deficiency in the functioning of vital organs. If water intake is neglected during fasting, up to 20% of liquids can be lost, which is usually fatal. This is why we emphasize the importance of continuous intake of liquids with a significant amount of electrolytes, which will enable the body to continue working normally, even if there is no direct intake of food and there is a transformation of stored energy into active and consumable energy.

Other physiological phenomena occurring during fasting

During intermittent fasting there are also other changes or phenomena in the physiological variables of the body. It is important to know them, because only by taking them into account will you know how to compensate for these variables, either through a diet rich in the elements that are lacking at a given moment or by avoiding those foods that could raise the levels of certain elements that are at their optimum point. Some of the components that can undergo changes are:

- **The leukocytes:** during the first days of fasting, leukocytes or white blood cells tend to rise. After almost a month of intermittent fasting, half or even less leukocytes are left compared to the first few days of intermittent fasting.
- **Red blood cells:** red blood cells increase steadily until the tenth day of fasting, after which they generally maintain their levels.
- **Plasma:** it is impossible to avoid a slight liquid loss in the

organism during the first days of fasting, since the amount of liquid coming from solid food is limited, and therefore, plasma tends to decrease during the first half of the month in which intermittent fasting was started.

- **Calcium:** it may drop slightly during the first months of fasting, although this does not happen in all cases.

CHAPTER V

Types of intermittent fasting

Fortunately, there are currently several types of intermittent fasts, each with a specific level of difficulty according to the goal you want to achieve. By choosing the ideal type of intermittent fasting, you can achieve great benefits from the beginning, starting with the main benefit, which is that your body gets used to the new diet. In addition to the new meal schedule that will be implemented, the body is also accustomed to weight loss, to the maintenance of an ideal weight and to many other benefits that we've already mentioned.

Next, you will learn about the types of intermittent fasting according to their difficulty, which are organized from least to greatest complexity. Thanks to them, you'll have success losing weight or improve other metabolic processes if you get to practice to the letter and following the timescales that are recommended.

Type 12/12 intermittent fasting
(*Time Restricted Feeding*)

Intermittent fasting 12/12 type is the easiest to perform and recommended for all those who begin to research the topic and want to accustom the body to a controlled food intake. This consists of fasting at the least 12 hours a day, which could be translated, for example, to implement the last food intake at 18 hours in the afternoon and not eating again until 6 in the morning the next day. That would be one way to fulfill the 12-hour fast. Now well, the second 12 of the equation are the times you can eat. For example, having the first meal (breakfast) at 6 am, the second at 12 noon and the third at 6 pm.

This intermittent fasting was one of the first to be analyzed through a study conducted with rodents in a controlled space. In the research, a group of rodents were fed low-quality fats and a large amount of carbohydrates for several weeks, in order to determine the effects of this diet on the species. The study concluded that the mice didn't just eat at night. As is normal in their species, but they also developed the habit of eating during the day, with the final consequence that they ended up rapidly developing problems of obesity, fatty liver and diabetes. However, that was not the highlight of the study. The experiment took an interesting turn when scientists divided mice into groups: those in the first group continued to be fed with the same unhealthy diet and food available at all times, while those in the second group were eliminated the possibility of eating during the day, supplying them the same foods as those of the first group but only at night.

The results were dramatic: those mice that ate during their natural activity did not develop obesity, diabetes or fatty liver, and even lowered their weight despite the diet being the same for both groups. What can be learned from the study? Simply, if you get used to 'snack' food at night for you sleep late you are driving your body to obesity, diabetes, heart problems and fatty liver. The good news is that you can eliminate this predisposition by practicing the 12/12 fast, which is nothing more than eating your three conventional meals during the day and resting at night.

Those who think that the results of this experiment do not apply to you are wrong. The staff who conducted the study with mice also selected a group of men and women volunteers were asked not only to stop eating at night, but also having breakfast a little later and dinner a little earlier. The results of this new study were just as surprising. After a few months, people had lost a lot of weight, have more energy to do your daily activities and a group before the study could not sleep went to bed go better and restorative way. And the truth is that this has a simple explanation: human beings, until a few centuries ago, only rested at night since there was not enough light to prepare meals and take snacks, leaving these activities for the next day when the sun lit up. That'd be why eating at night is relatively new to the human race and their metabolism is not ready to process all the calories and fat from the meals during these hours.

16/8 intermittent fasting: the starting point for a healthy life

The first type of fasting, rather than an intermittent one could be understood as a "return to normality", it's meant to adapt the body to the way it expects to act. So to say, basically eating only when there is sunlight, nonetheless the 16/8 type fast -spending 16 hours fasting and eating three meals in an 8-hour space during the day- is already beginning to accustom the body to a healthy diet.

To practice this fasting, you should simply fit your three meals in spaces of 8 and 8 hours, making sure that there is always light naturally. For example, have breakfast at 10 a.m., lunch at 2 p.m. and dinner at 6 p.m. before dark. In total, from 10 a.m. to 6 p.m., eight hours will have elapsed and you will have eaten three times with sunlight. While the previous fasting type of 12/12 eliminated the bad habit of eating at night, with this fast of 16/8 hours you begin to make your body adjust to a healthy feeding regimen (in terms of hours). In this way, you will not only maintain your weight and avoid related ailments, but you will also invite your body to start feeding on its fat stores. In other words, autophagy will start to kick in. And you may be wondering: «Why exactly 16 hours…? ». The answer is clear: because our body's glycogen stores are replenished every day with the meals we eat, which last approximately 15 or 16 hours. Therefore, in the 16/8 fast your body will be forced to use them during the early morning and another part later in it, because they do not receive any other food.

Eat-Stop-Eat intermittent fasting

This type of intermittent fasting is already considered demanding, so it should be practiced only when one has been practicing other less intense fasts for several months, such as 16/8 or 12/12. It lies on the fact that this fast consists of eating once a day, as simple as that. You may be thinking that it is impossible to eat only once a day and continue to perform in all your daily activities, but the truth is that there are people who take very good advantage of it because they do not restrict themselves at all during the only meal they eat per day. That is to say, they replace the abundance of a single daily meal with several small meals. When practicing Eat-Stop-Eat fasting, it is essential that the dish consumed be abundant in carbohydrates, proteins and good fats so that it serves as fuel for the entire day. The schedule of this meal is not restricted at all, since the person who practices it can decide if he/she prefers to eat breakfast, lunch or dinner.

Semi-fasting type intermittent fasting
(*Fasting Mimicking Diet*)

Although it is not specifically a fast, since it allows eating at any time of the day, the so-called semi-fast (or Fasting Mimicking Diet) takes into account the amount of food that is eaten. The semi-fasting diet consists of consuming 1100 to 1200 kilocalories for two days a week and then continuing for another four or five days with a diet that is around 700 or 800 kilocalories. The semi-fast is well regarded for loss of weight and to improve the health in a short time, but two things are essential: first of all, that people who practice it maintain a moderate intake of carbohydrates and, secondly, they have experience in other less rigorous fasting modalities. Fulfilling both points minimizes the probabilities of suffering decompensations and that insidious sensation of frequent hunger

5:2 Fasting

This is a diet that, although it is rather flexible, also requires practical experience with fasting, since it involves restricting food drastically for two days a week (ingesting only 500 kilocalories), and practicing any intermittent fasting mode for the remaining five days. "Very flexible and Comfortable!" you'll think, but the truth is that eating normally –or on a less demanding variant of intermittent fasting- for five days, would make the two days a week of intense fasting become a pain if your body is not used to it.

The best thing about 5:2 fasting is that, although it seems lax, it will allow you to lose weight and lower your cholesterol and blood glucose levels. There are even those who have tried to stop fasting for the remaining five days (eating healthy, of course) and have achieved these same benefits. It all really depends on the goal you have in mind. If you are not in a hurry to lose a few pounds, but prefer to do it little by little, you can practice the 5:2 variant where the only days you fast are the two mandatory days. Now, if what you want is to lose weight quickly and also get to improve your health in time record, you can combine this fast with other types of less demanding fast as 12/12 or 16/8. Remember not to exaggerate at any time when doing this fast (such as, for example, consuming 500 kilocalories several days a week) since you could end up weighing down your health and your body in a significant way.

The benefits of this type of fasting, in addition to the reduction of blood sugar and cholesterol levels already mentioned, include an improvement in the insulin sensitivity of the digestive system. This means that any food eaten will be processed in its entirety, retaining the vast majority of its nutrients. Also, with 5:2 fasting you will be directly preventing type 2 diabetes, which can arise from low insulin sensitivity. Partly because of this and partly because it can also decrease the amount of fats in the blood, this type of fasting is more advisable than a traditional diet.

Flexibility is another of its characteristics, because with the 5:2 fasting it will not be necessary to set just one or two meals a day, but you can set several meals that in total provide you with 500 kilocalories. In other words, you can eat as many times as you want per day, as long as you control the amount of calories that these meals represent in total.

The Warrior diet

Do not be confused by the name, since the Warrior Diet is actually a very powerful type of intermittent fasting, not a diet in the classic sense. The Warrior Diet was a creation of Ori Hofmekler, former member of the Special Operations in Israel and an expert in the world of nutrition, fitness and healthy lifestyle. Hofmekler explains that this diet mimics directly the diet that is supposed warriors and hunters of old followed, so it requires a lot of experience performing fasts that are increasingly demanding. Generally speaking, following the Warrior Diet you will not eat until you "get another food source" or, in other words, you will only eat once a day.

Another main condition for this diet is that the only food that is eaten in a day must take place during the hours of the night, in order to avoid the sensation of appetite before sleeping (a sensation that can make anyone sleepless). In addition, it is necessary that all foods are fresh, so say goodbye to canned and processed foods. You will have to cook! The foods that the expert recommends the most to follow this diet, which is considered the perfect intermittent fasting to lose weight quickly, are nuts, legumes, fine meats, vegetables and greens. To make sure that they are as fresh as required by the diet, we recommend that you shop at food fairs and traditional markets, places where there is usually a good influx of buyers and the product is replenished several times a week, which guarantees its freshness.

You may be wondering how you can eat just once a day without feeling hungry or weak. As we mentioned earlier in the eBook, the secret is not only in fresh, quality food, but also in liquids and natural juices. You can drink green natural juices (of cucumber, celery and cabbage, for example), lemon juice diluted with honey or juices of ginger, spinach, watermelon and blueberries. In addition, you can always drink coffee, tea and water, so you don't have to have an empty stomach during fasting hours. These drinks will act as the fuel your body needs and will help you lose weight, as each of the recommended ingredients has diuretic and antioxidant properties that contribute to fat loss. And you want to know the best part? All these drinks boost the feeling of satiety! You won't have to go hungry during this period by practicing the Warrior Diet.

Is the Warrior Diet really worth it?

We know that it takes a lot of effort to put up with the urge to eat several times a day, which is why we would not recommend the Warrior Diet if it wasn't such an effective diet. In fact, experts in the

Queen's Medical Center in Nottingham found that after a period of a few months practicing this diet metabolism increased to 14%. This helped each of the people who practiced it in processing properly the fat of consumed foods, which stopped them staying in the body and as such the glucose was used immediately.

However, what has not yet been proven is whether or not this intermittent fasting is sustainable. And everything points to the fact that it will depend primarily on the health status of the person who follows it (health comes first) and their willpower. Normally we recommend that, apart from the Warrior Diet, once you have reached your ideal weight according to your height, you migrate to a less rigorous intermittent fasting that ensures the maintenance of said weight.

24-hour intermittent fasting

Surprise! There was still a type of intermittent fasting to mention, which is nothing more and nothing less than total abstinence from food. During a 24-hour fast, you can only drink water, tea, coffee, and other calorie-free drinks or juices. To practice it, you can only have one meal a day, which may be lunch. After this, you can only eat again for lunch the next day. This type of commonly fasting combined with intermittent fasting of type 12/12 16/8 or 5:2, so it may be practiced on one day of the week.

In fact, due to its characteristics, the practice of this type of fast is delicate, because if you are not completely used to fasting, you will experience different sensations as a consequence of being for a whole day without eating. Among them, irritability, excessive appetite, weakness, dizziness and possible fainting, therefore it is absolutely necessary to have practiced fasts of type 12/12, 16/8 or 5:2 before intersperse your week a day of fasting for 24 hours. Now well, the truth is that when the person is used to it, the advantages of this fast are notorious: your body will purify a great amount of fats, completely emptying a great part of the reserves lodged in different areas of your body, your metabolism will improve, insulin will work better at the moment of processing food and your blood sugar level will go down, among other benefits.

CHAPTER VI

What can you drink during your fast?

Although we have discussed above some juices and drinks that can be taken during intermittent fasting, this chapter will expand this information to the max. By doing so, we hope that by the time you finish a period of fasting, you won't wonder why you didn't lose weight if you stopped eating one or two meals. Because, indeed, there is little or no use in fasting in terms of food for a certain period if you do not give up Coca-Cola or other sugary drinks, for example. The good news is that even though soda and other sugary drinks are not allowed, you will be able to drink other liquids besides water, which many people don't know. So no, you won't be enslaved to a glass of water. You are about to discover which drinks are recommended during intermittent fasting and, in the case of juices, how to prepare them so that they are delicious and also have diuretic effects, burn fat and keep you satiated between meals.

Drinks you can have during intermittent fasting

There is a large variety of beverages taken during this period of fasting, either during the stage start, in which the body gets used to the fast, be it in the beginning phase, in which the body is fully used to the period of starvation or low number of calories to be supplied.

Infusions

Infusions are very popular beverages that, apart from quenching thirst, have innumerable health benefits because they are extracted from ingredients that come from nature. Infusions are composed exactly of chemical elements from the extracts of leaves, fruits and stems of certain plants. However, they rarely come ready-made, instead they have to be put in hot water (infused) so that the disintegrated and dehydrated organic matter leaves its components in the water, thus offering us a very nutritious and tasty beverage that is usually drunk hot.

Did you think that Coca-Cola and other carbonated beverages in general are the most consumed in the world? Well, no, this position belongs to mineral water (which we will talk about later), followed by herbal teas. The main reason why herbal teas are so popular is not only because they are delicious, but also because, being the product of organic matter sources, they can help prevent different diseases and even cure them. These properties have been known since ancient times and today their effectiveness is still intact. There are different types of infusions that you can take during fasting periods. These will reduce the probability of hunger and keep you hydrated and nourished during this period.

Tea, without a doubt, is the most popular herbal tea in the world. Originally created in China, it was initially taken only for medicinal purposes. Precisely for this reason, most of the population could not drink this infusion, since it was provided as an advanced treatment against various diseases such as colds. Only royalty, nobles and wealthy families could try it. However, during the 16th century it started to become a popular drink simply because it was so delicious. There are many types of tea around the world, but the most consumed are the five main types: black, green, red, white and blue tea, being green the most widespread. Some of the characteristics of each variety are as follows:

- **Black tea** has one of the strongest flavors in the world of teas due to the oxidation process to which it is subjected. It has a good amount of caffeine, so it could replace coffee in the morning. This is, along with green tea, one of the most consumed types of tea in Asia.
- **Green tea**, the most commonly consumed in Asia, usually comes in sachets with dried leaves. It comes directly from the *Camellia Sinensis* plant, in Latin, which is a rich source of antioxidants in the form of polyphenols.
- **Red tea** is one of the finest tea drinks there are. For it to be ready for consumption, it can take from one year to more than sixty years. This happens because the red tea plant goes

through a fermentation process that is critical for its final flavor, typically mannered and with a very characteristic aroma.

- **White tea** is very soft and has an exquisite aroma. It is made by taking the upper leaves of *Camellia Sinensis*, the same plant that produces green tea, and letting by helping them wither naturally.
- **Blue tea**, finally, also called 'Oolong' tea is not a single type of tea, but includes several subtypes of blue teas. All of them have a touch soft, but there are some with floral flavors, tastes that are slightly stronger or more oxidized.

The benefits of tea are multiple and well known: it has anti-inflammatory and antioxidant properties and its consumption can help burn fat. But when drinking tea, it is important to take into account its origin, because although tea in its natural state is excellent for the body, there are products and brands to which sugar is added or are not stored properly, so look for quality teas.

As for coffee, it needs no introduction. It is consumed worldwide and many people drink it every day to start the day thanks to its high amounts of caffeine, which help the body to activate. In the West, for example, it is the most consumed beverage after water. Coffee is obtained from the beans of the coffee tree, drying and grinding each one of them until they are powdered. Normally, its taste is quite bitter if no sugar is added, so it is recommended to drink it not too concentrated, as it is not recommended to add sugar during strict intermittent fasting. However, if you are one of those who cannot drink your cup of coffee without sweetening, you can use some 100% natural resources to sweeten it, such as honey.

Another of the best known infusions -which is not necessarily the most consumed- is mate. Mate is a type of infusion that is obtained by cutting and heating the leaves of the mate tree. Like coffee, this plant is cut, dried and ground until the organic matter is obtained, which is placed in a small cloth bag destined to be inserted into the cup, where this delicious infusion will be taken. Mate is somewhat acidic, so other herbs with a milder flavor are usually added to enliven it or honey to sweeten it. It is an infusion widely taken in Argentina and Uruguay. Besides being very tasty, mate contains a large amount of antioxidants that prevent premature aging of cells and prevent both cancer and heart disease. Like coffee, it also has energizing properties to keep you active throughout the day.

Sodas with low or no sugar content

"How!? Can I drink sodas during intermittent fasting? », You will be asking yourself. Our answer is simple: yes, but in moderation and as long as they are sugar-free. The truth is that light or zero soft drinks do not contain sugars and can be consumed from time to time throughout the week. But what we should certainly not do is to accustom the body to the consumption of these drinks, because at any time your usual supplier will stop having the light or zero drinks and, as you have gotten used to them, you will end up asking for a traditional one with plenty of sugar.

It would be best not to have them during intermittent fasting, but eventually, if it does not contain sugars, there is no harm. However, the reality is that, unlike all the drinks we have mentioned before, sodas lack of positive contributions for your diet beyond taste. They are just liquid candy, so it would be best to avoid them as much as possible. Now, it is obvious that between not drinking liquids and having to drink a diet soda, we encourage you to drink the soda, since staying hydrated during your intermittent fasting period is absolutely necessary to avoid decompensation.

The importance of hydrating with water

Hydrating with water is essential while fasting. Water will 'occupy' the stomach while one of the meals of the day arrives, but the truth is that it has a more important function: it will keep you properly hydrated, reducing the risk of decompensation. Keeping yourself hydrated with water will not only be more economical than opting for herbal teas or sodas; it also has different benefits, including the following:

- **It will prevent you from having headaches:** in case you didn't already know, if you have a frequent headache, it may be due to moderate dehydration. Drink water frequently!
- **It will help your digestive system:** the metabolism may be slower in the absence of water. However, if you have water in the stomach at the time of digestion, this will take place normal-

ly faster if you had not drunk water.

•	**It will reduce the chances of heart problems:** you should drink up to two liters of water daily to reduce the likelihood of heart attacks and even diabetes. Water will help improve your circulation, replenish lost fluids and help vital organs function better.

•	**Lose extra weight:** Undoubtedly, one of the main advantages of drinking water is that you will lose extra weight. The explanation is simple: when we drink water, it takes the place that food should occupy in the stomach, achieving a feeling of satiated appetite and thus helping to maintain fasting for longer. In addition, because water has no carbohydrates, sugars or fats, it is perfect to replace the sweets or sodas that are taken between meals.

•	**It will eliminate fatigue and weakness:** water is perfect to eliminate any weakness that may occur during the first few days of fasting. In fact, it is possible that when you feel weakness is due to the lack of moisture, so it is recommended that you drink some water anytime that happens.

CHAPTER VII

Diabetes and intermittent fasting: compatible?

You may be concerned about your pre-diabetic or type 1 or 2 diabetic status when it comes to intermittent fasting. This is a logical concern, since fasting will affect your metabolism, blood sugar levels and energy reserves, but fortunately this type of fasting is recommended for diabetics and there are few points against it. In any case, first of all it is advisable to know how to differentiate the three types of diabetes that exist:

- **Gestational diabetes,** which can occur at approximately 5 months of pregnancy, even if the mother has not been predisposed to diabetes before. This is a type of diabetes that must be treated to prevent the death of the baby.
- **Type 1 diabetes**, which mainly affects children and young people, although it can also be diagnosed in adults, with a small percentage of cases falling into the latter category. Type 1 diabetes occurs when the body's defenses destroy the pancreas, since the person is no longer able to produce insulin, a substance that is absolutely necessary for the cells to absorb nutrients from food.
- **Type 2 diabetes**, which occurs mostly in adults. It is a diabetes that can be prevented more easily than type 1 diabetes if intermittent fasting and exercise are combined, since its cause is obesity and sedentary life. In this type of diabetes the pancreas can produce some insulin, but not enough to process all the food that enters the body.

Once the different types of diabetes are known, it goes without saying that the chapter will only address type 1 and type 2 diabetes, as intermittent fasting should be left to the discretion of a physician if performed by a person with gestational diabetes. Either way, in all cases of diabetes, we recommend consult ar first with one medical specialist applying a meal plan through intermittent fasting. The difference is noticeable and can help you choose a type of fast based on your health and diabetes.

Intermittent fasting and type 1 diabetes

Intermittent fasting can be a blessing for people with diabetes of any type, as it improves insulin action and lowers blood sugar levels. However, there is one thing that anyone with diabetes who wants to lose a few pounds should keep in mind: blood glucose levels will change as soon as any type of intermittent fasting is started. And this change in blood glucose levels will make it necessary to adjust the amount of insulin being given. If a person neglects this aspect and begins intermittent fasting without the advice of an endocrinologist or nutritionist, it can result in the insulin dose being higher than necessary, leading to a high glucose burn in the body and hypoglycemia. In other words: a drop in glucose and possible dizziness, fatigue and even fainting.

It is advisable, especially in cases of type 1 diabetes, to monitor glucose levels during the first months of fasting so that you can know how your body is reacting to the new feeding system. In this way, you will stay one step ahead of your diabetes and control any abnormal insulin and blood glucose levels. The normal thing to do when visiting the doctor in case you want to start an intermittent fasting diet is that the professional invites you to measure your insulin levels as you progress with fasting. This is the only way to determine whether or not it is necessary to eliminate a certain dose of insulin from your daily routine, exactly the same insulin that your body would use to process a meal that you are going to skip, for example. Another idea that your doctor could also suggest is the use of long-acting insulin or, if you already use it, your doctor could recommend reducing its use by up to 50% as the intermittent fasting process progresses.

Intermittent fasting and type 2 diabetes

In the case of type 2 diabetes, just the opposite happens than with type 1 diabetes, since it has been found that it is contra-productive to deprive the body of food when you have it, according to studies by the Salt Lake Research Unit of the Intermountain Medical Center Heart Institute in the United States. The researchers suggest that people who practice intermittent fasting to improve their type 2 diabetic condition should immediately stop their practice, as it can make type 2 diabetes worse. Intermittent fasting is contraindicated, they say, mainly because it causes the amount of glucose to fall or rise beyond normal and/or treatment-controlled limits, which is called glycemic variability. Although this tends to appear mainly in type 1 diabetics, in type 2 diabetics this glycemic variability oscillates strongly reacting to a caloric restriction coming from fasting.

High variability in blood glucose levels produces a number of side effects, which is the main reason why intermittent fasting is contraindicated for this group of people. These side effects may include retinopathy, coronary heart disease, weakness and dizziness. However, such effects could be avoided by choosing a fixed type of intermittent fasting and, in case you wish to change it someday, you should go back to the endocrinologist or nutritionist to fix a new diet suitable for intermittent fasting. In any case, if you decide to practice this diet with type 2 diabetes and medical control -or even if you are still not very clear about your position on the matter-, we are going to list the advantages and disadvantages of intermittent fasting with type 2 diabetes.

Advantages of intermittent fasting with type 2 diabetes

As with caloric restriction diets (which can be of different types), there are also many types of intermittent fasting. Therefore, if you have diabetes, you can choose the one that best suits your health condition and, once you have selected the most comfortable type of fasting, you simply have to follow it and monitor its results in terms of weight and in terms of blood glucose levels. This last aspect is essential because knowing the blood glucose levels produced by a certain type of intermittent fasting means that there will no longer be a wide glycemic variability. You will always eat at a specific time or times during the day, so you will not need the same dose of insulin that you have been injecting, but a lower one because there are fewer nutrients to metabolize.

You won't have to count calories

While in a diet you have to count calories for the three, five or six meals you eat each day, in intermittent fasting you won't have to count calories (although you will have to use common sense to avoid foods or beverages that are harmful to your diabetes and weight). In intermittent fasting, the work of calorie restriction is done by the reduction of one, two or three meals a day (depending on the number of times you currently eat per day, including snacking and between-meal snacks). And usually a restriction of one meal leaves you more satisfied than restricting the calories of all the meals of the day, something that usually leaves a feeling of appetite that is difficult to get rid of. So the first advantage of intermittent fasting with type 2 diabetes is that you can eat as much as you want in one or two healthy meals a day without having to count calories.

It is effective in controlling blood sugar levels

This may be a somewhat controversial aspect depending on the researchers, but the truth is that studies conducted by Dr. Suleiman Furml with a group of volunteers in 2018 determined that even intermittent fasting can be the ultimate solution to not having to inject insulin frequently as insulin levels are always controlled.

Dangers or Disadvantages of Intermittent Fasting with Type 2 Diabetes

Actually, there is only one notorious disadvantage to intermittent fasting with type 2 diabetes, namely, uncontrolled default blood glucose levels. As for the rest, it is true that there are other general disadvantages, but they are not unique to fasting with type 2 diabetes, but can commonly be associated with both intermittent fasting and any dieting regimen.

There is a lack of glycemic control

As we have already mentioned, blood glucose levels will alter with any intermittent fasting. They may go up or down in comparison with the normal blood glucose range, which is the result of the usual insulin treatment provided to all diabetics. But this can be solved by monitoring your blood glucose levels.

The process of adapting to intermittent fasting will be more difficult

During the adaptation process, which usually lasts between one and two months, you may feel confused, because you used to know when your insulin injections were due and your body was familiar with both the treatment and the subsequent blood glucose levels. However, the moment you start fasting everything will be different because you will have to adapt to the new schedule or diet and remember when your new insulin doses are due. In some cases, you will even have to cut out some of the doses you are used to taking. Most often, since it is all a matter of adjusting, after the second month you will have your lifestyle under control and you will be completely adapted to intermittent fasting.

You may feel a bigger appetite and eat more during your next meal.

Perhaps the most difficult challenge you may face as a diabetic in the process of adapting to intermittent fasting is to eat more or less the same amount of food at every meal and every day. Therefore, portions may be somewhat larger than when you were on a simple calorie-suppressing diet, as hunger is something you will not be able to avoid. Due to this common circumstance, your blood glucose levels may be out of control during the first months of adaptation. We recommend that you visit your endocrinologist for ideas on how to reduce the anxiety produced by skipping a meal, although you can also follow our tips to 'entertain' your stomach while the next meal arrives.

Can intermittent fasting help in case of diabetes risk?

The experience of some diabetics with intermittent fasting has not been good. Blogger Rosy Yanez, for example, says that in her experience she achieved a perfect balance by fasting in the mornings and eating more in the afternoon period, something she did because "during the mornings blood glucose levels rise naturally, so it is better to eat in the afternoons the first meal of the day". However, Yáñez also states that "each person is different, so you should choose a type of intermittent fasting that is perfectly adapted to each type of organism and normal glucose levels" since there can always be imbalances in the plan. According to the blogger, "during the first few weeks I felt the need to increase food portions in the next two meals of the day, which I regulated as my body got used to fasting". Although the most striking aspect of Yáñez's experience is that, according to her, the days when it was more difficult for her to skip a meal were the days of menstruation, when, due to the hormonal imbalance, she had a greater sensation of appetite and anxiety to eat.

Now, although the blogger's experience may not have been

as satisfactory as she imagined, the advantages of fasting according to her testimony are clear: you will not have to look for a breakfast according to a low glucose level to avoid a glycemic disorder, but you can simply skip it, achieving a natural balance of blood glucose. It can also be concluded, according to their testimonials, that it decreases the inflammation typical in people with this disease, improves their blood pressure and insulin does its job more effectively. This means that, although there may be a lack of glycemic control when a person with diabetes practices this diet, it is also true that people with diabetes can control it by attending a visit to an endocrinologist and nutritionist.

Reasons why intermittent fasting works for type 2 diabetes

There is a resistance to insulin in type 2 diabetes, and this is responsible for carrying the glucose found in the blood to the cells to feed them. However, in the absence of a normal level of insulin in the blood, it is not possible for insulin to control the full amount of glucose that is also in the blood. After developing the predisposition to diabetes, which is normally diagnosed when there is a very high level of glucose in the blood that insulin is not being able to handle, then comes the diagnosis of type 2 diabetes as such, which is when there is insulin doing its job (carrying glucose to the cells) but in such a high quantity that, once it is in the cells, it spills out because there is too much in the organism.

What is most interesting is that treatment with extra insulin in type 2 diabetes can worsen the problem of excess glucose in the blood. The explanation is simple: yes, there will be more 'transport' (insulin) for the 'passengers' (glucose), but the destination of those passengers will be a crowded place where they do not fit anymore and therefore have to leave (thus returning the glucose to the blood). What then is the ultimate solution? There are up to three solutions that we are going to explain. The first is exercise, through which you can burn excess body fat (which, remember, is stored glucose to be used later). A healthy lifestyle with moderate exercise is essential.

The second solution is to eat a reduced-calorie diet and the third is to simply prevent more glucose from entering the body than the body needs, which can be achieved by intermittent fasting. Quite a few people have successfully eliminated type 2 diabetes from their body by following intermittent fasting, which allowed them to control the excess glucose in their body. When the excess glucose is eliminated and glucose enters the normal range, a full life can be lived, thanks in large part to intermittent fasting.

CHAPTER VIII

Fasting and the brain

So what does fasting have to do with the brain? Aren't we talking about losing weight and body fat? Clearly yes, but intermittent fasting is a whole box of surprises, since in addition to the benefits we have already explained, it can help us stay young both in terms of mental sharpness and external appearance. This is directly related to the process of autophagy, the 'art of eating oneself', which, although it has nothing to do with cannibalism, is perhaps a bit similar since the body begins to feed on its own energy reserves in the form of fats or free radical cells by not giving it food. In addition, since the digestive system rests thanks to intermittent fasting, other areas of the body such as the brain can function optimally, achieving greater concentration and performance.

Evolution, Intermittent Fasting, and the Brain

Studies focused on the evolution of both humans and other mammals have found interesting points that can give us details of what is really important for the continuity of a species. For example, studies have shown that if a member of a species is deprived of food for prolonged periods of time, certain organs in its body are likely to shrink, except for the brain and the reproductive apparatus.

This is explained by the fact that the brain needs to be used to stay alive and survive the potentially dangerous situations of everyday life, but it is also necessary for the reproductive system to be intact (in the case of males) so that they can procreate and maintain the species. So forget about your mind being 'foggy' while fasting due to the absence of a meal (since the opposite will happen) and don't worry about your ability to reproduce either. This has a logical evolutionary explanation: if food is scarce, a weak mind would be a big problem, since it would make it even more difficult to get food, so the body sends energy directly to the brain. In fact, testimonies of soldiers who were imprisoned during World War II reinforce this logical theory. They stated that while locked up they had moments of lucidity in which they were able to perform activities at a higher rate than normal in the realm of learning.

However, the cognitive benefits of fasting go beyond increased attention and ability to concentrate. Tests on rodents have yielded very surprising results in terms of motor skills, memory and the ability to learn new skills or habits. The differential of this study is that it was carried out with elderly mice divided into two groups, one of which was fasted while the other group was allowed to eat freely 24 hours a day. The result was that those in the first group, the mice subjected to intermittent fasting, showed a lower propensity to Parkinson's disease and Alzheimer's disease. This is easily explained by the fact that a specific protein, BDNF or Brain Derived Neurotrophic Factor, is activated in the brain when low levels of nutrients are detected. This protein has the important task of sending orders to neurons that interact directly with the area dedicated to learning, memory and cognitive functions that act in some mammals and humans. When the levels of this protein are low, predisposition to Alzheimer's disease, depression and various learning and concentration problems may appear.

Intermittent fasting helps to progressively raise BDNF protein levels, which positively affects the field of memory and Alzheimer's prevention, prevents depression, learning ability deterioration and neuron death. Now, the best thing is that in our brain there is another protein that has a similar function as the BDNF protein: GDF11. It protects our brain from premature aging by creating new neuronal networks and blood vessels in the brain. Although this hormone is normally found in mammals and younger humans, it began to be seen at higher concentrations in people and older mammals once both began to practice intermittent fasting. This means that the brain of an older person can begin to recover from aging when the body is deprived of one or two meals a day for an extended period of time.

CHAPTER IX

Fasting and the heart

Heart disease is an unfortunate trend in today's world. No matter what part of the world is given as an example, you can see these types of diseases (among which the most common are hypertension, heart failure and cardiomyopathy). However, and despite how widespread they are, what many unfortunately do not know is that they may be sabotaging their heart health through what they eat and drink. One of the main risk factors is certainly high cholesterol levels in the blood, as it makes it much easier to develop heart disease, heart attacks and strokes. Thus, cholesterol in all its manifestations is considered a serious problem for the body if its levels rise beyond normal. Since cholesterol has only half-deserved fame, in this chapter we will refute the widespread belief that all cholesterol is bad, which is not true.

First of all, cholesterol is necessary for the human body, both because it exists in the body by default and because it has the important job of creating several groups of hormones and repairing cell walls in case they have been damaged. The cholesterol that takes care of these essential processes is known as 'good cholesterol', while bad cholesterol is the product of a poor diet and is responsible for causing various diseases to develop. The good news is that nowadays we can know the levels of both, since there are laboratory tests that can determine the values of good and bad cholesterol. The process is simple: good cholesterol is measured with a high-density lipoprotein test, while bad cholesterol is measured by examining low-density lipoproteins. It is important to know that when a high cholesterol level is determined, it is specifically talking about low-density cholesterol, as it is the high levels that will affect your health.

This condition can be successfully treated with medication, but it tends to return within a few months because in many cases we are not treating what caused the high levels, but rather the main symptom. To attack the root of the problem it is necessary to know what caused it; although there are many hypotheses, it is believed that the main reason for high cholesterol is an inadequate and unhealthy diet, characterized by fast food, a poor nutritional balance and the frequent consumption of sugary foods. However, the truth is that there is another interesting fact that you probably did not know: what happens to fat when it has been stored in the liver for a long time waiting to be processed? This fat is converted into a substance known as triglycerides, which is also related to a rise in low-density cholesterol levels. Moreover, when this glycogen leaves the liver converted into triglycerides it creates a major problem. In a patient who has, for example, a high range of bad cholesterol and whose triglycerides are elevated, the attention of professionals will immediately turn to evaluating the value of the latter, since they are much more harmful than the bad cholesterol itself. In any case, you must be clear at all times that storing fat is counterproductive to the health of your heart, which is why it is necessary to eliminate it with intermittent fasting!

Triglycerides play a major role in causing cardiac arrest, stroke, or the beginning of chronic heart disease, so it is a value that we must be very aware of in order to preserve our health. In fact, triglyceride levels are one of the statistics that has increased uncontrollably for more than five decades in countries with a high consumption of junk food (United States, for example) compared to other disease statistics, such as type 2 diabetes or obesity. To treat high triglycerides it is advisable to follow a low-carbohydrate diet, which works very well both to reduce these values and to reduce the rate at which the liver creates them. However, to avoid low-density cholesterol this solution is not entirely effective.

Surprise! Bad cholesterol does not solely depend on nutrition

For decades, our trusted doctors have recommended us to avoid foods that contain a considerable amount of fat and cholesterol, as this would effectively prevent our cholesterol levels from rising. Have you ever heard the famous phrase "eat low-fat and low-cholesterol"? Well, that is precisely what has always been recommended, since "the lower the level of foods with high cholesterol, the lower the risk that this value increases in the body".

But the truth is that if you already have a high level of cholesterol in your body, a low cholesterol diet will not help you to eliminate the one that is already unbalanced in your body. This has been recently discovered by the scientific community, from which it was believed since 1913 that cholesterol, being a component that clogs the arteries and usually results in a fulminant heart attack could be reduced in these areas of the body if you simply consumed foods that had less cholesterol. This approach was taken for granted from that time until today, when it has been studied and disproved. The truth is that, although eating little cholesterol does reduce the level of bad cholesterol in the blood, the levels at which it is reduced are negligible. When this belief was widely accepted, a group of scientists led by Nikolai Anichkov conducted an experiment in which they fed a rabbit with a high amount of cholesterol, causing arteriosclerosis. Thanks to this experiment, it was determined that consuming cholesterol caused a blockage in the joints. However, there is a very curious fact that nobody noticed, although it is very logical: rabbits are not really prepared to process cholesterol, since in their natural environment they only eat plants, which have little or no fat.

It was not until the 1950s that the effects of a high-cholesterol diet on humans were studied by Ancel Keys. Keys gathered a group of people with different eating habits, weights and percentages of body fat, among other of the dividing features he applied, and conducted a study consisting of administering foods with a very high amount of bad cholesterol to see if they increased the levels of low-density cholesterol in the blood. To the researcher's own surprise, feeding the chosen subjects in this way did not raise their blood cholesterol levels. After that, not satisfied with the result, he expanded the range of the experiment to seven other countries and obtained identical conclusions: he had discovered something very important for people's general health! There was, however, a big question... What was causing the high cholesterol levels in the blood? Scientists quickly found a possible cause: dietary fat. After several years of research, however, they concluded that it was not the responsible factor, as they found no hard evidence to point to it as such.In fact, this same research yielded a surprising result: the more fat, the less cholesterol in the blood, which further complicated matters for the researchers, who wanted to prove just the opposite.

However, this group of scientists proved to have a warrior soul, since none of them was willing to communicate the results of their research to the world until it was what they were looking for. Thus, in one of their last attempts, they invited volunteers to undergo two types of diets: one low in fat and the other with a high fat content. Again, the surprise for them soon followed. After several months on these diets, they discovered that the percentage of low-density cholesterol in the bodies of the volunteers in both groups was... the same! Indeed, all the volunteers in group A and all those in group B had the same cholesterol level with which they started the study, respectively. Moreover, the difference between groups (despite the very opposite diet they had followed) was almost non-existent. The result that was closest to the one they wanted to test was, of course, for the group of people who increased their intake of cholesterol-rich foods by a large amount, but the difference was only 4 points between the beginning and the end of the 50-day experiment.

Once again, however, the scientific community of the time did not readily accept the results of this experiment, so low cholesterol and low-fat intake continued to be recommended to avoid high levels of bad cholesterol in the blood. It was not until 1977 that a different nutritional recommendation was introduced and adopted in the United Kingdom and the United States. This stated that a low carbohydrate intake should be recommended in order to "prevent heart disease", which is false and carries an immediate risk, as demonstrated in 1983 by Zoe Hardcombe. So, knowing as we do today that a low-fat, low-cholesterol diet does not prevent heart disease or other unfortunate health episodes... So, what should be done?

Intermittent fasting as a definitive method for lowering cholesterol

The main cholesterol-producing organ in the human body is the liver, where it is produced in order to carry out the metabolic processes of the organism in which this compound is necessary. Now, what happens when you consume less cholesterol than usual (which was advised by scientists in the last century) is that the liver notices the low amount of carbohydrates in the blood and begins to produce more of them. Thus, eating fewer carbohydrates invites your body to produce more to cover its deficit.

It has finally been shown that just two months of fasting could help the body eliminate up to 25% of bad cholesterol, which means that intermittent fasting would be more effective than a total of 50 days of low-calorie, low-cholesterol, low-fat diet, as recommended in the past. It is true, however, that intermittent fasting is 50% less effective than conventional medical treatment, but its advantage is that it is completely natural. Fasting reduces the production of cholesterol by the liver as it will produce less triglycerides as it perceives fewer carbohydrates. It is key to remember that excess cholesterol is immediately converted into triglycerides, which directly affect the heart and other vital organs, so it can be concluded that intermittent fasting will help you preserve the health of your heart.

In fact, triglycerides are the precursors of bad cholesterol and their absence lowers cholesterol levels. Studies have found that intermittent fasting for about 70 days will help the body reduce low-density cholesterol by up to a quarter of the total amount in the body and reduce triglycerides by a third of the total amount. So what's the good news? The first is that skipping one or two meals a day intermittently can have the same effect as a rigorous low-calorie diet, approaching the results you would get through medication, with the advantage that intermittent fasting is totally free and easy to do. And now you must be thinking: "What's the second good news... Why not start with drugs or low-carb diets if they have the same effect as intermittent fasting? Quite simply: intermittent fasting, while it is true to say that it has similar effects on cholesterol control as drugs or diets, has the benefit of reducing your weight without reducing lean fat. In other words, with intermittent fasting you will reduce bad cholesterol without reducing good cholesterol and, of course, you will reduce the risk of suffering from cardiovascular diseases or diseases such as Alzheimer's disease.

CHAPTER X

Fasting and exercise

It is normal when recommending a sports diet that it is heavy on carbohydrates to stay well-nourished and avoid fasting to arrive at a training or competition. However, there is a major problem with diets based on carbohydrates, and that is that these are stored in very little proportion in the body, while fats are stored in abundance. In our body there are several fat deposits, which have the function of preventing us from dying as a result of a lack of energy, which the organs need to function normally. But such fat is present in such a quantity (especially if you have a few extra kilos) that it not only guarantees that you can live for several days without food, but also allows great efforts. For example, a runner can run several laps of a stadium without stopping for a day before his energy is consumed in the form of fat.

The perfect solution for the body to not only feed on carbohydrates, but also on stored fat in the form of glycogen, is to do periods of intermittent fasting, with which the body can be forced to use reserve energy when it cannot find carbohydrates to digest immediately. It is a way to burn fat, not get fat and be active. However, there are certain considerations to take into account, such as the intensity of the sport being practiced. In normal cases, the body reserves fat for times when it needs to exercise under a high-intensity regime, burning these reserves to allow the body to have enough energy to move at high speed or withstand long days of physical activity. But if glycogen is depleted during low-intensity workouts, sponsored by intermittent fasting, this can affect high-intensity exercise. This is why it is necessary to understand the essential functioning of our body in the face of an exercise regimen, which is exactly what we will see in the next point.

The body and its energy system

The body is a large machine in which thousands of natural processes are carried out in order to keep it functioning properly. One of these vital processes for energy to flow between muscles, nervous system and organs is the production of adenosine triphosphate (ATP), a component that enables cells to fluidly draw energy from fat and other parts of the body. The energy catalyst ATP is stored in every muscle; however, when training or engaging in a high-performance sport activity it can be consumed in a matter of seconds, leaving the muscle without its usual energy-absorbing capacity. Fortunately, there are three ways to return this catalyst to normal levels:

- **Through the phosphagen system.** There is a component in the muscles called creatine phosphate, which is responsible for creating new ATP. However, phosphagen is found in the muscle in very small quantities, so it can generate new ATP only during a few seconds of sporting activity.
- **By the glycolytic method.** This ATP replenishment system works by using the glycogen stored in the muscles. It is the second route of ATP production, although this process also releases the lactate hormone, which generates the sensation of fatigue. Although it is capable of producing ATP for minutes at a time, it is not sufficient for a day of continuous activity, such as a soccer match, a day of crossfit or a light jog for hours.
- **Through the aerobic system.** Finally, there is the aerobic system, the optimal method for creating ATP. Normally, the aerobic system only begins to function when ATP production by phosphagen and glycogen is exhausted, thus giving way to fat burning. Fat burning occurs because ATP is produced directly from the mitochondria by this system (which requires oxygen), and this process consumes large amounts of fatty acids or what is the same, conventional fat that is stored in our body. In fact, there is so much fat to feed the aerobic ATP production system that we could walk for days without falling to the ground.

Thus, it can be concluded that in order to perform sports activities it is necessary that the aerobic system is activated, allowing the process of using fats and glycogen. We should remember that glycogen is recharged thanks to the carbohydrates in the food, while fats are the energy surplus that the body does not need at the moment, so it stores them for later use in case of food shortage. It is also interesting to know that all the lactate that is produced in the glycolytic system is also immediately utilized by the body, since it is converted into glucose by metabolic processes. Now that all these concepts are clear, it is time to debunk the myths about intermittent fasting that we have blindly believed over the years, which are as follows.

You'll lose strength if you don't eat every meal of the day.
It is commonly believed that if you do not eat every meal of the day, including the occasional snack, your body can lose strength and power, two attributes necessary for running at high speed or lifting weights, so you don't want to lose just these abilities in the middle of a workout or competition. Do you? Well, this is just a myth, since both muscle strength and power depend on phosphocreatine, a protein that is not affected by skipping one or two meals a day. In fact, it has even been proven in competitions that practicing intermittent fasting does not affect the body's strength or power levels. Proof of this was a study conducted by the International Society of Sports Nutrition, which found that intermittent fasting for 30 days for a group of professional gymnasts did not affect their strength at all compared to other athletes who did not follow the regimen. Moreover, most surprisingly, the gymnasts did not lose strength, but they did lose fat.

If I practice intermittent fasting I will lose muscle mass.
This is one of the most popular myths about fasting, since it seems logical to think that if the muscles do not receive enough carbohydrates during the day they will end up losing volume. However, this is not the case, since the volume is maintained, what may be more difficult is to acquire a greater muscle mass than you already have or define muscle from scratch, although it is worth emphasizing that for these goals a specific diet for muscle gain or definition is necessary and intermittent fasting seeks to reduce the levels of fat in the body.

So, if you are determined to gain muscle it is better to go for a diet rich in carbohydrates, but if you want to lose fat while toning your body (after all, it is healthier to control the index of body fat), then we recommend intermittent fasting. Now, in the case of body-builders or weightlifters, eating a diet with intermittent fasting will not affect the level of strength and power.

Fat burning only occurs thanks to aerobic system training.
Given that fat burning starts in the body's aerobic process, you may think that glycogen is not needed in the body, but this is not the case. While the body's energy stores are activated after several minutes of high-performance exercise, glycogen is responsible for providing the body with enough energy to move from a resting state to the new state of fat burning in exchange for energy. In fact, glycogen stores are so important that, when the time comes for fat burning thanks to the aerobic process, fat burning is prioritized over the use of glycogen, so it will be possible to save this protein when starting the aerobic process to obtain ATP and you will not feel tired after passing to the resting state.

Can I combine intermittent fasting with exercise to lose weight?

When you talk about losing weight immediately, two alternatives may come to mind: doing it with a low-calorie diet or doing exercise routines to activate the body's aerobic system so that it can start burning fat. But the truth is that there is, of course, a third option, which is intermittent fasting. This brings us to the question of whether it is possible to combine intermittent fasting with days of exercise, since in addition to processing fat to function, our body would be benefiting from the additional fat loss that the aerobic system would burn. So can fasting and exercise be combined? The answer is yes, although it depends on the type of exercise you are going to do. Because if you are in the middle of training to increase muscle mass, the results may not be as optimal as they would be with the high-fat, high-carbohydrate diet. However, if your goal is to lose body fat, weight and improve your overall health, the combination of sport and intermittent fasting will work for you.

Thus, intermittent fasting is recommended for people whose

main goal is weight loss and even muscle toning. And the perfect exercises for this are those of low or medium intensity, such as squats, light running, sit-ups or push-ups, among others that do not require a great effort for a long time. But what if you want to gain a lot of muscle mass, endurance and at the same time lose weight and improve your health? Intermittent fasting can also help in these cases as long as the training sessions are not too long (3 to 5 hours a day) or you train at different times (for example, in the morning and in the evenings). The reason for this is that it is very difficult to ingest the necessary calories from a hypercaloric diet in only one or two meals a day, so the results in terms of muscle gain will not be as good as those that can be obtained with a hyper-caloric diet.

When is it best to exercise while fasting?

There are different types of intermittent fasting and different types of exercises, although nutritionists recommend doing workouts after 14 hours. The reason for this is that after the workout the appetite may be triggered and, if the workout takes place in the morning and it was planned to fast during those hours, it will be very difficult to avoid the consequent hunger. However, this does not take away another alternative recommendation of the experts, which is that if the person is training for a high-intensity sporting event, the intake should take place two or three hours after the event in order to take advantage of both the nutrients in the food and the glycogen and fatty acid deposits, thus obtaining more energy.

Essential food when you exercise while fasting

Eating a healthy diet is absolutely necessary when practicing intermittent fasting, but it is even more so when you start fasting while practicing high-impact training or moderate exercise. There are foods that in addition to being healthy can provide high levels of energy for both your day-to-day life and for training. The so-called healthy 'superfoods' for athletes are the following:

- **Rice.** Rice is an ingredient that is included in a good part of the dishes we eat throughout the month, but if you are still not very used to eating rice, you better reconsider, as it is an important source of energy thanks to starch. In addition, it can supply the body with an important dose of vitamin B, it's very low in fat and high in fiber, making it easily digestible.
- **Sweet potatoes.** Sweet potatoes are another special food that should not be left out, especially if you are an athlete and practice intermittent fasting. This ingredient will bring a remarkable amount of energy to athletes due to its generous amount of iron and will fight high cholesterol and high blood pressure problems.
- **Lentils.** Lentils are an exceptional food that is not only recommended for athletes, but for anyone who practices fasting. The reason is that by consuming just a handful of lentils you will feel a prolonged feeling of satiety that will help you meet the goal of skipping a meal a day. But the main reason is that eating lentils will provide you with a large amount of folic acid, iron, vitamin B6, manganese and potassium.
- **Olives and avocados.** They are necessary ingredients in any diet since they provide healthy fats to the organism, as well as a generous amount of iron, folic acid, potassium, magnesium, iodine, calcium and vitamins A and B groups.
- **Eggs.** Eggs are essential in any diet, even more so for those who practice intermittent fasting. They provide the body with unsaturated fats, which are good fats, promoting the increase of good cholesterol. It is also low in calories and high in protein, so it will help keep your stomach fuller for longer, and it is free of artificial preservatives.
- **Vegetables.** Whether steamed or raw, vegetables should be present in any type of diet because they provide an immense amount of nutrients in exchange for very few carbohydrates. We have broccoli as an example, which is an excellent source of vitamins, proteins and minerals with very low percentages of fat that can regulate abnormal levels of glucose in the blood.
- **Meats.** Meats are necessary for a daily diet as they are full of proteins, responsible for replenishing muscles after any high

intensity training session. In addition, meat consumption promotes good cerebral oxygenation and provides the body with high levels of hemoglobin.

With these ingredients you can create different incredibly tasty and healthy dishes, as is the case of the *Poke Bowl*, an original dish from Hawaii that includes several of the ingredients that we have mentioned and can raise your energy levels before or after training, all without getting fat and without having to cut out the ingredients you like the most from your meals! Of course, these ingredients considered *superfoods* are essential, but microfoods are also necessary and include all those that belong in the fruit and nuts group in order to complement the diet in the training process.

Contraindications when fasting and practicing sports

Nutrition specialists agree that it is essential to familiarize the body with the absence of one meal a day before training, exercising or jumping on the court to practice any discipline. This recommendation seeks to avoid dizziness, weakness or possible fainting that are typical during the first weeks of fasting. That is why it is key to take it into account before starting an intermittent fasting routine and jumping into sports without thinking twice. After about three weeks practicing intermittent fasting, you can begin low-impact sports routines, with which we will gradually transition into more demanding ones. But, in any case, the key to success is to get the body used to it first and then move on to the exercise routines that you were already doing before practicing intermittent fasting.

CHAPTER XI

Intermittent fasting in women

Men and women tend to have different goals when fasting; although this is determined by a number of people surveyed and does not mean that this is always the case. What is certain is that women mostly seek to lose weight using intermittent fasting, while men focus more on muscle growth and loss of body fat index. As we have already addressed in the previous point the case in which most men fit, we will do it now of the characteristics, advantages and disadvantages of intermittent fasting in women, especially focused on weight loss. We will tell you that the main advantage of intermittent fasting is that it is incredibly flexible, because you can adjust its intensity and it will always give you good results if you do not fall into the habit of snacking on junk food between meals as before. Above all, you must have willpower!

We also warn you that intermittent fasting can alter metabolic processes specific to women's bodies, such as the menstrual cycle, the onset of menopause or metabolic disorders, and the latter especially in young women, who are those with high levels of hormones. Understanding these disadvantages as a starting point, it is necessary to approach intermittent fasting in a controlled manner, accustoming the body to the new diet.

Is intermittent fasting healthy on a hormonal level for women?

With intermittent fasting, as we have already mentioned, women's hormonal cycles may be affected, something that will last until the body gets used to the new dietary regimen and the new schedule proposed for it. The most affected area will undoubtedly be the menstrual area, where the hormones GnRH, LH and FHS act, all of which control the reproductive processes in both men and women. Because the ovulation process in women is especially sensitive to hormonal changes, they can be significantly affected in their ovulation cycle. This can occur if you start with a cycle of intermittent fasting that is too tough to start the new lifestyle. Because, although it is necessary to lose weight, it is even better and more necessary to properly ground the fasting foundation so that your new lifestyle does not collapse soon after due to starvation. Rigorous intermittent fasting can significantly unbalance menstruation, causing it to be delayed or to occur prematurely.

In addition to this recommendation, it is necessary to consider your level of hormonal sensitivity. Women who are more hormonally sensitive should incorporate intermittent fasting slowly into their daily routine, allowing fewer hours of fasting and devoting a little more time to the process in which the body gets used to it. For example, for hormonally sensitive women, the recommended fasts are the 5:2 and 16/8, already studied, which will not represent too much effort or change in eating patterns, but still leave important health benefits. After a few months following them, if you fit in this case, you can try to change to a more rigorous fast if you want to lose weight faster, but the change should be equally gradual.

Should I avoid intermittent fasting as a woman?

Only in some specific cases that we will address below is it advisable to avoid intermittent fasting. In case you fall into any of them, it would be best to suspend intermittent fasting and consult a nutritionist for advice on the best alternative to lose weight safely.

Avoid intermittent fasting if you are pregnant
Intermittent fasting should be avoided during pregnancy, as it drains the body's stored energy in the form of fat and problems can arise during pregnancy and fetal nutrition (let's not forget that there are two organisms that must be fed). Intermittent fasting is known to improve cellular responses, decrease predisposition to diabetes and

can also provide increased energy, but these benefits are not applicable during pregnancy. Why? Because during this period the nutrient and vitamin levels that the fetus receives will depend directly on the mother's good nutrition, so the pregnant woman will have to eat whenever she is hungry to benefit both the growth of the fetus and her own energy gain.

Avoid intermittent fasting if you plan to become a mother.
A woman's fertile response can be affected if intermittent fasting is practiced as a lifestyle, especially in women over the age of 25. In fact, failing to practice intermittent fasting in a correct way can trigger a hormonal response that ends up accelerating a menopause or causing infertility. It is, therefore, highly recommended for women in their fertile stage and with any difficulty to conceive -current or past- to consult with their trusted physician to find a healthy alternative to lose weight (which can be intermittent fasting, but always under the endorsement of a physician). In such cases, reducing the amount of carbohydrates, but not the number of meals per day, is an appropriate alternative. In other words, if you were already doing intermittent fasting and now you are planning to get pregnant, it is a good idea to follow a calorie - restricted diet.

If you are underweight, intermittent fasting is not advisable
Intermittent fasting, as you know, focuses primarily on reducing body fat and weight. Therefore, by adopting a regime of intermittent fasting you will assimilate glucose better and detoxify the body, among other benefits that we have already covered, but at the same time you will lose even more weight. And that, in cases where the starting weight is already low in itself, will be counterproductive to health. Now, if you are only about 3 or 5 kilos lighter and you want to benefit momentarily from some of the benefits of fasting, you can do so, but always for a specific amount of time. If the weight imbalance is greater than a 5 kg deficit, you need to consider other methods to achieve your goals, as it will not be healthy for you to continue losing weight.

Intermittent fasting, women, and diabetes
If fasting as a woman already has a number of important considerations, diabetes must also be taken into account, and women must be extra vigilant in this regard. In addition to the hormonal imbalance

that occurs in women as a result of intermittent fasting, insulin levels can drop or shoot up depending on factors as diverse as the type of fasting practiced, the time of the meal that is avoided or ingested and the times at which insulin doses are administered. Therefore, it is absolutely necessary to keep track of insulin levels throughout the day if you want to practice this fasting, without forgetting the opinion of an endocrinologist who can interpret each glucose and insulin level constantly. An alternative, as in the case of pregnant women, is to practice a reduced-calorie diet that avoids extra pounds and keeps cholesterol and insulin levels stable.

Women with eating disorder and fasting

Eating disorders occur more commonly in women than in men, these are important diseases that affect health due to strong negative emotions, so they are also related to mental health. People suffering from eating disorders have problems to eat properly because they believe that whatever they eat will deform their figure. Therefore, they decide not to eat or they eat and moments later vomit so that the fats are not stored in the body (anorexia and bulimia).

If a family member has anorexia or bulimia, among other eating disorders that may occur, or is recovering from them, it is not advisable to practice intermittent fasting, as they may try to cover up (even involuntarily) their disorder, making it look like a completely natural activity that brings benefits. If you are the one who is going through or has gone through such a disorder and do not have family support, you should be honest with yourself and ask, "Am I covering up my eating disorder by intermittent fasting?" Many women with this type of disorder practice intermittent fasting to validate their disorder, both for themselves and for family and friends, which will affect their health even more.

To avoid covering up an eating disorder it is necessary to thoroughly follow each of the indications that we give you in this eBook, among which the most important is not to skip more meals than those suggested in each of the types of intermittent fasting and, of course, to gradually move from a less rigorous type of fasting to a harder one.

We also suggest you to tell a family member about your fasting plan and have them assist you in monitoring your progress, for which you will need to be completely honest with them.

So, should women fast?

Fasting is not recommended for both genders -especially for women- when there are very specific illnesses or situations, such as those already stated. In any case, if there is only a problem of overweight, you are not breastfeeding, you do not have an extremely low weight or problems of eating disorders or diseases that require large amounts of energy reserves for recovery, it is advisable to fast. Nevertheless, it is always smart to make an appointment with a health professional so that he/she can give you the necessary approval, recommend the best type of intermittent fasting according to your conditions and possible future fasts to which you can switch to once you get used to introductory fasts.

CHAPTER XII

Men and intermittent fasting

Men usually combine intermittent fasting with some sporting activity to help them lose weight at a fast pace, but mostly to gain muscle in the process. And that's even knowing that intermittent fasting is not the optimal training plan when it comes to gaining muscle quickly (it is effective, yes, but there are diets that guarantee faster results). However, this last unfavorable point can be compensated by eating a large amount of good quality calories at each meal of the day and avoiding heavy carbohydrate intakes in the evening if you do not plan to exercise.

Combined with a good eating plan rich in carbohydrates the high-carb diet recommended for people who are training for any sporting activity can be equaled and even surpassed, since the bene-fit of intermittent fasting is that it will allow you to lose weight while developing your muscle, so you 'kill two birds with one stone'. Of course, as we have been saying, it is necessary to eat large meals to get the amount of carbohydrates needed, although with the help of a nutritionist you will be able to plan an appropriate diet for your in-termittent fasting in training phases. In addition, you should take the pressure off yourself, because during the first months of intermittent fasting you do not need such a high carbohydrate intake, since you need to lose some weight to start toning the muscle in question. Therefore, you will need to consume high-calorie dishes only as your demand grows, thus achieving both muscle toning and muscle gain, which is what many men desire.

In the case you feel very tired, we recommend implement-ing periods of rest between exercises because when forcing the body (even more during the first weeks of fasting) you can cause damage to muscle tissue and lead to frustration. To ensure that the muscle recovers properly, especially during the first weeks of exercise, it is necessary to ensure a high protein intake in your meals of the day.

What if I am not interested in gaining muscle but in losing weight?

If you want to go step by step and lose a good amount of weight as you progress with intermittent fasting, you can focus on progressing through the difficulties of fasting, going from 5:2 to 16/8 and so on, until you achieve your ideal weight or a close one. Once you are at that point, you can decide whether to complement the fast with low or high intensity exercise routines, for which you will have to increase the amount of daily carbs.

Intermittent fasting and testosterone: you should increase your levels

It still is not 100% proven, but apparently intermittent fasting can increment a little the testosterone levels, which is the hormone involved with fast production of muscle mass, with sexual desire and increased stature thanks to the hormonal growth. But, in addition, testosterone has the power to help repair tissues affected by exercise routines, which turns fasting into a powerful tool to optimize muscle gain and weight loss, among other interesting aspects if you are a man.

CHAPTER XIII

Foods to eat after the fasting period (and breaking it)

Thinking about what foods to eat after a period of fasting is an interesting topic since the body (as it has been out of the food processing for a while), will optimally process the next meal you eat after fasting, which means that you can process very well both healthy meals and meals in which saturated fats abound. That is why, after 24 or even 36 hours of fasting, you should think carefully about what foods you can break the fast with in order to take advantage of all the vitamins and avoid an upset stomach. The following tips will help you decide the first daily intake after fasting, avoiding any kind of problems and improving your health.

Hydration is vital

Both during and after fasting, hydration is vital, but when breaking the fast, it is important to first ingest liquids that maintain a good level of mineral salts, so that your body can carry out the digestion process in a fast and effective way. In addition, it is advantageous to break the fast with liquids to prepare the digestive system for the imminent ingestion of solid food. And when we say liquids, it means that you can even prepare a tasty coffee or tea with a little milk, which in small quantities does no harm (on the contrary, it prepares the stomach for the reception of food).

Breaking the fast with solid foods gradually

After this brief liquid based introduction it's time for solid foods, but, as your stomach might have not received food for more than one day, you should be careful. At the least, if you want to avoid an upset stomach or the digestive system from absorbing poor quality fats, bad cholesterol or large amounts of sugar or sodium. Why is it necessary to eat gradually and not to gorge or eat conventional meals after a fast? Because there will be an absence of digestive enzymes in the stomach, which are not produced at the same rate as a day ago because the body assumes that they are not very necessary at the moment. Therefore, if more food enters the body, the digestion process may not proceed normally. The amount of digestive enzymes is not enough and it is necessary to readjust the digestive system to solid food. If you do not gradually make this transition and eat normally, you are likely to suffer from episodes of diarrhea, undigested food and, in rare cases, vomiting and dizziness.

Types of Foods That Work Great for Breaking the Fast

There are different foods that are easily digestible and guarantee the absence of digestive problems. Some of them are salads and white meats:

- **Salads.** Salads should be prepared with cooked vegetables to avoid adverse reactions. You can add raw cucumber to the salad (this ingredient can go uncooked because it is a fruit), tomato and parsley, as well as a little avocado.
- **White meats.** Together with salad (or even in it) you can add chicken breast, which is an important source of protein. Although besides chicken, other white meats such as fish are also recommended. Since these white meats have little fat, olive oil is recommended to improve the flavor or to cook them.

Foods and drinks that you should not consider to break the fast

Foods that can be harmful to the digestive system are those difficult to digest due to their composition, as well as others that may have a high degree of acidity. Some of these foods not recommended to break a fast but which are widely consumed are alcohol, milk, cheese, eggs, seeds, dry fruits and red meats (although sometimes they may be consumed without problems in low quantities). It is important to remember that, in addition to avoiding these foods as much as possible, you will have to wait about six hours after breaking the fast to be able to eat in normal portions. In this way, you ensure that the digestive system produces the necessary enzymes to process food normally.

What happens if I accidentally drink alcohol to break my fast?

In the case of consuming alcohol things get a little more dangerous, as consuming alcohol after several hours of not eating can lead to alcoholic ketoacidosis, which appears when alcohol is consumed with low blood sugar, a scenario that can occur when performing intermittent fasting. Low blood sugar levels can be further affected by high levels of alcohol, leading to severe stomach pains or vomiting in mild cases and dizziness in some more severe cases.

Refeeding syndrome after fasting

Occasionally, eating again after a period of a day or more of fasting can cause severe symptoms such as fainting, heart failure and even coma. This is known as refeeding syndrome, produced by a large movement of electrolytes in people with low levels of potassium, calcium and magnesium in the blood, levels that can become low during prolonged fasting. During fasting, the body enters a state of reserved energy consumption, in which magnesium, calcium, potassium and phosphorus are also consumed. Just when the body decides to reactivate the digestive system to process the food that has recently reached the stomach, these ions are also required to reach the cells so that a normal hormonal function can take place in order to process the energies. But these are insufficient to cover all the cellular demand, which triggers this syndrome, with which the following symptoms may occur:

- Seizures
- High blood pressure.
- Confusion.
- Weakness.
- Fatigue.
- Cardiac arrhythmia.
- Coma.
- Death.

Risk factors for Refeeding syndrome

The reality is that thanks to the progressive evolution of the food sector, almost nobody has to hunt to be able to eat nowadays. Rather, it is necessary to have money, to shop in a supermarket and to cook. We are therefore all much closer to overeating than to malnutrition, but this first factor can also have a significant impact on our health, especially when we come out of a period of malnutrition or a long period of fasting. You are more likely, in short, to be affected by refeeding syndrome if you meet some of the following characteristics at an organic level:

- You have an eating disorder.
- You consume alcohol frequently.
- You are undergoing chemotherapy.

- You're on insulin treatment.
- Your levels of phosphorus, magnesium, calcium or potassium are very low.
- You have fasted for more than four days on liquids alone.
- Your body mass index is less than 18.5%.

How do you avoid refeeding syndrome after heavy fasting?

This dangerous syndrome, although not so common, should be avoided as much as possible. In addition, to avoid it you only have to consider some simple to follow precautions:
- Avoid eating large amounts of food to break your fast.
- The first meal should not be high in carbs.
- Drink plenty of fluids every fasting day. Choose drinks and juices rich in electrolytes and with very low or no sugar content.
- It is necessary to salt your meals, even if it is in small proportion.
- Try not to fast for more than 3 days. In case you need to fast for a longer period of time, medical supervision will be necessary.

In short, as you can see, there is no need to worry about refeeding syndrome if you have not eaten for less than 24 hours. In fact, there should be no problem with 36-hour fasts if you are at a good weight and eating well. What you should do is eat healthy, low-carbohydrate foods high in good fats and easy to digest. If you follow all our advice, it will only be necessary to plan in detail with what ingredients you will break the fast when the time comes and as long as it lasts for more than 24 or 36 hours.

CHAPTER XIV

Tips to adopt intermittent fasting in your life

When practicing intermittent fasting, as in other areas in life, consistency is needed to achieve the desired results. Intermittent fasting works in a similar way to dieting: if you do not follow the routine in your everyday life, you will return to the same weight you had before. The main advantage of intermittent fasting is, as you know, that you can eat a normal amount of calories and carbohydrates in each of the meals of the day (unlike those diets in which they are restricted), suppressing - however - at least one meal. Many people will think that it is difficult to get used to it, but actually, from the third week of intermittent fasting this new diet will be something completely natural for you. What is true is that, while you reach that stage, it will be necessary to put your body through a process of getting used to the new 'rules', so it is necessary to follow the following tips to adopt intermittent fasting in your life.

Choose the right fasting plan

We mention this first of all because the main reason why people who start this type of fasting give up is because they do not choose the right type of intermittent fasting. In the eagerness to lose weight quickly, some people tend to choose intermittent fasting with a level of difficulty that, as beginners, they will not be able to sustain over time. That is, they may be able to practice strict fasting for a week or two, but this lifestyle will not be sustainable and will end up generating a feeling of failure. This could be the case of a person who chooses a fasting type of 6 days of normal food and one day only based on liquids, where normal food is eaten one day and the next day a limited amount of calories is eaten, usually around 500 or 700.

Therefore, both nutrition experts and people who have already practiced intermittent fasting and adopted it as a regime of hours between meals recommend starting with an undemanding fast, such as 5:2 or 16/8 at the most. These diets, although they will not make you lose weight overnight, will get your body used to new, more demanding intermittent fasts, which are the ones that can make you lose weight quickly while cleansing your body.

Don't rush, your body will let you know when it's ready

Another common mistake is to move from one style of fasting to a more demanding one too quickly. Although both studies and the experience of people who practice this fasting indicates that the body gets used to it between the third and fourth week, it does not mean that you have to change the fasting you have been practicing. The transition to the next more demanding type of fasting should be slow, accustoming the body to the new scale of difficulty. This can be achieved by moving further and further away from the new plate of food as the days go by, thus moving from a 5:2 diet to a 5:3 diet and finally adopting another type of diet such as the 16/8 diet, which represents the next immediate level of difficulty.

If you feel that hunger is uncontrollable or, in rare cases, you feel weakness and dizziness, it will be convenient for you to resume the previous type of fasting while you gradually adjust the difficulty of the next level. How can you make this progressive adjustment? Well, for example, by eating one hour later than you usually do or by eating only two meals instead of the four or five meals you normally eat daily.

Get used to doing everything in stages

There are different stages for the organism to adapt to fasting. There are usually seven main stages through which you will establish the pillars of your new dietary conception. These seven phases that you must follow are the following:

The detox phase

This phase begins the moment you decide to start intermittent fasting and lasts until your body gets used to the complete elimination of processed foods. It lasts approximately four days, in which you must say goodbye to fast food and all the pre-processed foods you used to eat. With this, the body will no longer be storing large amounts of fat as before, and you will have taken the necessary step to start burning the excess fat. For several days you should eat home-cooked meals with at least 50% carbohydrates, 20% good fats and 30% protein.

This phase is related to 5:2 fasting, as it is the first intermittent fasting that nutritionists usually recommend to those who start. Given the coincidence, you should eat for five days only homemade food with the balance we recommend and then spend two days eating 3 to 2 times a day with a very low amount of calories. Do not forget to hydrate very well during these two days of fasting!

The high protein and high fat phase

During this phase you will be able to eat a high amount of protein and unsaturated fats, that is, good fats. This phase begins when the body has already become accustomed to the absence of processed foods and fast food, so you will be able to balance your food at 40% good fats, 40% protein and 20% carbohydrates. Obviously, cooked vegetables will be your best ally, which you can serve with fruits such as sweet potatoes, tomatoes or watermelon, as long as you eat them as part of the main course and not as a dessert. Sometimes it is preferable to leave fruits for breakfast, as well as natural yogurt, since they are not recommended for the rest of the day (especially in the afternoon and evening). And, of course, sweets are forbidden unless they are from natural ingredients.

The hydrate phase

The third phase is the carbohydrate phase, in which you can take a break from the usual rigor of intermittent fasting. This phase is usually practiced twice a month (the second and third week for a maximum of four days) in order to make the fast a little more flexible. It is important to note, in any case, that the carbohydrate phase does not mean that intermittent fasting will be broken and you can eat fast food with carbonated drinks, but rather that you will only get to eat a few more carbohydrates than usual. More specifically, you can eat up to 40% carbohydrates, 20% fat and 40% protein, so that the carbohydrates are doubled compared to the immediately preceding phase. A good idea to take advantage of this week is to eat fruit for dessert about twice a day (in company, therefore, with every meal) and a fruit as a snack in the afternoon/evening.

As you can deduce, the heavy meals recommended for this diet are those that contain a good amount of carbohydrates, such as rice, potatoes, pumpkin, quinoa, lentils, beans, oats and nuts, to name a few examples. All of them also have a good percentage of healthy fats, so they are ideal in phase three, although if you are not completely convinced and you are still not satisfied with the flexibility of fasting in terms of ingredients, you should know that you can also eat chocolate. Of course, the chocolate must have 70% cocoa (the healthiest) and the limit will be half a bar a day.

In the variety lies the secret

The key to not getting bored of dieting or intermittent fasting is, without a doubt, variety. Variety in your diet will help you achieve a better balance between ingredients and, of course, the benefit of not getting bored of always eating the same thing. In previous chapters we have indicated various ingredients and combinations so that you can eat in a healthy way, therefore you should combine them in ways that you enjoy, ensuring that they provide exactly the amount of protein, good fats and carbohydrates that we recommend. Over time you will see that not only will you be progressing in your adaptation to intermittent fasting, but you will find the process very easy, so add variety to each of the three meals of the day!

Drink liquids to replace meals

One of the things that helps people the most in their process of adapting to fasting is to drink liquids instead of eating solid foods. For example, if you are someone who is used to eating constantly for almost the entire day, you can start to eliminate those meals or reduce the amount of calories in them. However, the very moment you do so, hunger will arrive, so a cup of tea, water or a small glass of natural fruit juice will allow you to replace it without the uncomfortable feeling of hunger (or at least it will mitigate it a lot).

Eat your last meal of the day in the late afternoon

On this point there are conflicting opinions as many recommend eating late at night, while others recommend not doing so, but we are going to explain to you the reason for each of the opinions. From a general point of view, eating late at night is always contraindicated, because from 9 pm onwards the processing of fat in the body will be inhibited because the body takes advantage of the nutrients of the food eaten late at night. It is also possible that reflux may appear, that phenomenon that occurs when stomach acids go from the stomach to the esophagus producing an unpleasant sensation of acidity. In addition, there is evidence that the carbohydrates you eat at night can be easily converted into fat, something that goes against the purpose of intermittent fasting, which is to lose weight.

From the second point of view, however, there are professionals who advise intermittent fasting by eating at night. They argue that it is perfectly possible to do so without negative side effects, for which they recommend doing exercise that leaves you exhausted before eating. With this, instead of being stored, the carbohydrates will tend to restore the cellular structure of your muscles, leaving them as good as new and thus enabling the option of eating at night without negative repercussions. However, this does not mean that you can eat any type of food at night. Fatty foods or foods too rich in carbohydrates are forbidden. Otherwise, it is recommended to eat at night all kinds of sweet potatoes (sweet potato, yucca and potatoes, among others) and a piece of fruit (banana is ideal).

We recommend that, if you can eat just before nightfall (later in the afternoon), do so, as this will prevent the carbohydrates in your meals from being transformed into fats if you are not practicing a day of exercise. Obviously, if you can't eat dinner in the afternoon then practice an exercise routine just before your evening meal and try to keep mealtimes short to avoid other annoying symptoms such as reflux or indigestion. Finally, remember that it is much better to opt for foods rich in protein rather than carbohydrates, as protein repairs your muscles while you sleep.

Failure is human

In the course of adapting to your new eating schedule, you may be overwhelmed and fail. Grabbing a snack or a fast food meal is something that can happen to anyone in this context, but it is essential that you don't get discouraged or give up because of it. You can let one, two or even three mistakes go by, but if you start to see that failing has become a daily routine it's time to apply some self-discipline. Let's suppose, for example, that you have been fasting for a week of 5:2 fasting and just on the day when you have to fast by eating very few calories you are invited to eat out, and not exactly healthy food. If you took that opportunity to enjoy with friends you must promise yourself that it will not happen again, unless you visit a restaurant where they serve light dishes. If this becomes a habit, you can discipline yourself by skipping the next meal of the day or fasting one more day a week.

It is highly advisable to keep this in mind so that you do not feel handcuffed to a new diet. Because in the end the goal is to make this new habit a norm in your life. So that you can motivate yourself and keep track of your process of adaptation to intermittent fasting, it is advisable that you design a calendar where you mark month by month the days in which you complied with the meals and adequate portions and the days in which you failed. You will see how this will encourage you not to fail.

Make comfort prevail

The last of our tips for normalizing intermittent fasting is to choose a type of fasting that allows you to be comfortable and fits into your day-to-day life. This is the only way to avoid seeing it as something that you find difficult to do or that requires a lot of discipline. Deep down you should understand it for what it is: a new healthy lifestyle that will allow you to lose weight or keep it off with very low percentages of fat and bad cholesterol. If you are about to give up intermittent fasting because it does not suit your reality, try a different one or something more flexible, but do not give it up, because you will lose the advanced and then you will have to start from scratch.

CHAPTER XV

The most popular myths about intermittent fasting and the practice of fasting

Over the centuries, a lot of myths have been created around the practice of fasting and others specifically about intermittent fasting. Today we are going to list each one of them and clarify whether they are true or not. You won't believe the number of myths about intermittent fasting that are just that: myths!

Myth1. Stop eating for a day? Impossible!

One of the main myths surrounding intermittent fasting in its most rigorous version is based on the belief that it is impossible to stop eating for a whole day without suffering negative repercussions on the body or on the performance of daily activities. But what none of the people who believe this yet know is that overeating is the trigger for obesity. The normal thing when inflating a balloon is that it increases its size due to the air; if this amount is excessive it ends up exploding or being very susceptible to explode in a short time. Well, something like this happens with the organism: when it is fed in excess, the rest of the nutrients are transformed into fat, making us put on weight. What intermittent fasting does is to use those extra fat reserves, which are the reserved fuel and... It deflates the balloon! Therefore, this myth is actually inconsistent, as fasting is a completely healthy practice if done in the progressive way that millions of people practice.

Myth 2. Fasting will cause the body to receive fewer nutrients!

To understand why intermittent fasting does not interfere with the amount of nutrients in the body, it is first necessary to know that there are two main types of nutrients: macro and micro. Macronutrients are fats, carbohydrates and proteins, while micronutrients are those that come in the form of vitamins and minerals. In intermittent fasting, the body is deprived of food for a normal period of less than 24 hours, so micronutrients are not affected and, in any case, if the fast reaches 36 hours (as some people eventually practice it), the lost micronutrients can be restored in a few meals on the day the fast is broken.

In the event that you do more rigid intermittent fasting, such as the Warrior Diet (among other fasts in which you spend more than a day or two fasting), consuming some multivitamin is recommended to avoid any nutrient deficits. This will not be necessary for the first months of fasting or in fasts that normally last less than 24 hours, since the body will be feeding on fats (macronutrients). During fasting, in addition, the body enters a state of reserve of micronutrients, which are normally lost through feces and urine, but during fasting the need to urinate and defecate decreases, so micronutrients can be better preserved. The body also performs, in order to ensure that nutrient levels remain stable, a process by which proteins are transformed into amino acids and then transformed back into recycled proteins. In cases of illness, pregnancy, lactation or recovery of any kind, we recommend that fasting should not be practiced since the body needs new proteins all the time, but we will see this topic in the next chapter.

Myth 3. Fasting leads to the need to eat more afterwards

Some traditional diets have a devastating rebound effect, whereby the cravings to eat something forbidden are so intense that you end up falling into them, eating large amounts of food (binge eating) and returning to the starting point with an even higher weight than when you started the diet. Fortunately, this does not happen with intermittent fasting, as the body will be used to skipping one or two meals a day after a process of adaptation. And the truth is that, although there is a small increase in the amount of calories eaten at each meal after starting the fast, these do not exceed the calories lost. That is to say, the amount of calories lost during the fasting day is higher than the amount of calories added to each plate of food during the day. If we add to this the fact that our experience indicates that the longer we fast, the less cravings we have for food, so the myth collapses by itself.

Myth 4. Fasting causes low blood sugar levels

Low blood sugar levels cause hypoglycemia, a condition that produces symptoms such as sudden dizziness, pale skin, weakness, trembling and excessive sweating. Hypoglycemia has been linked to periods of prolonged fasting, but you should know that, in the case of intermittent fasting, it is not possible for it to appear. Sugar levels are very important for the body and the body has a variety of methods to monitor them. By not receiving food at the time it is normally consumed, the body begins to take energy from the glycogen contained in the liver to generate glucose. This process usually occurs when fasting, but it also occurs every day while sleeping to ensure that sugar levels are adequate in the body, even if food is not received. Momentary glycogen reserves can be used up after 24 hours of fasting, after which the liver is forced to generate more glycogen through the process of glycogenesis. This is why fasting does not actually cause low blood sugar levels.

Another myth that is often related to glucose levels and brain function is the belief that the brain is only fueled by glucose, which is why people tend to have difficulty concentrating and thinking critically during fasting, which is not true. The brain uses glucose to function, it is true, but it also feeds on ketones, which are produced when fat is metabolized. In other words: while the body burns stored fat (thanks to fasting) it is also possible for the brain to remain in a perfect state of functioning, because in the absence of glucose from meals it starts the process of fat burning and the production of ketone bodies, which go to the brain cells to be fed.

CHAPTER XVI

Who should not fast?

Intermittent fasting must be taken seriously and be well defined. This ensures that the weight loss is sustainable and does not affect your health in a negative way. And, while it should always be taken seriously, there are certain scenarios in which intermittent fasting simply cannot be practiced for the sake of health. We've already looked at some of them, but let's dig a little deeper and find out why.

Nursing mothers

We know that after pregnancy you will be very anxious to lose the extra pounds you have gained during this period, but it is convenient to wait. The breastfeeding baby acquires all the nutrients it needs from its mother. Thus, if the mother has a small deficit of micronutrients, something very typical of intermittent fasting practiced for a long time, the baby will not be able to absorb them throughout its development since the remaining nutrients in the mother will be used by her to meet the needs of her body. If the baby does not receive the necessary nutrients during this period, its growth may be affected, since breastfeeding is vital in the acquisition of calcium, minerals and vitamins necessary for its bones and organs to grow in a healthy way. Fortunately, the breastfeeding period usually lasts less than a year, so at the end you can resume your intermittent fasting to lose the pounds you gained during pregnancy.

Pregnant women

As with breastfeeding, the vitamins and minerals present in the pregnant mother's body are the only food the fetus has to grow and develop properly. During pregnancy, it is vital to supply the fetus with as many nutrients as possible to avoid genetic abnormalities or health problems in its growth. In fact, many women do not produce an optimal level of nutrients and therefore must take supplemental vitamins to ensure the proper development of the fetus. Among these supplements that should be consumed is folic acid, an essential vitamin whose deficiency can cause defects in the brain or nervous system. So, at least during the 9 months of pregnancy and the months of breastfeeding, you should stay away from intermittent fasting.

Complications of type 1 diabetes

As we have already indicated in the corresponding section, if you have diabetes it is advisable to visit an endocrinologist to assess your health condition, your blood sugar levels and your glucose production before starting any fasting. Why? Because with fasting you will be modifying your eating habits and consequently your glucose values and insulin production may vary. And a change in these levels can cause health problems or unfavorable symptoms that affect your lifestyle.

You are very underweight

Intermittent fasting helps you lose weight by burning stored fat in your body, which is then converted into usable energy. However, if you are already at an already low weight, you may not have enough stored energy for your body to function autonomously for 24 hours or less. The central risk of practicing this fasting when your weight is low is that, if your body fat level is less than 4%, the body will not only process the fat, but also the protein, thus carrying out the so-called wasting (the progressive deterioration and extinction by combustion of the muscle). This process will be eliminating the muscular mass, among other functional tissues of the organism, so that it can continue to function with the hope of obtaining food soon.

As we know, the average body fat index is 25% in the case of men and 30% in the case of women. You may be thinking: "It is very difficult for someone to reach 4%". The truth, however, is that this index of 4% is actually the limit of what is risky when it comes to intermittent fasting, because in that range your life could be at stake. That is why it is recommended not to perform intermittent fasting if the body fat index is less than 20%, since the reserves can run out very quickly in certain circumstances. Also, keep in mind that if you are underweight or have a standard weight with a body fat index of less than 20%, under no circumstances do we recommend prolonged fasting (meaning fasting for more than 24 hours or for too many months).

Children and teenagers

Children and teenagers are exempt from the practice of intermittent fasting since during these two stages the body will be forming and requires a high concentration of vitamins and minerals for physical growth and the development of the brain and cognitive abilities. Intermittent fasting at this stage could inhibit the development of different parts of the body, as they need an excellent amount of nutrients to be able to function while developing. The most drastic and direct consequence of intermittent fasting in children or teenagers is therefore malnutrition. The only case in which intermittent fasting in children or teenagers is permissible is when it is carried out in a sporadic, controlled manner and never lasts longer than 24 hours.

People suffering from reflux disease (GERD)

Gastro esophageal reflux, or GERD, is nothing more or less than the heartburn experienced sooner or later by people who eat at night or at late hours. It is the typical sensation experienced when stomach acid has refluxed back into the esophagus. Reflux thus affects the tissues of the throat and generates a feeling of discomfort in the stomach. This problem appears especially in people with a good amount of fat in the abdominal region, which presses on the stomach and causes the acids to rise up into the esophagus. And if intermittent fasting is practiced with this risk factor, the heartburn problem may worsen, since there will be no food to keep the acids in the stomach. A solution to reflux could be to place your head and trunk at an incline that does not allow acids to rise to this area, but if you notice that the problem persists, intermittent fasting is strongly discouraged.

Conclusions

As you have seen in the eBook based on data and evidence, intermittent fasting has a wide margin of success in making anyone lose weight and body fat while accelerating your metabolism, among other important health benefits. We have outlined each and every case in which intermittent fasting is recommended, as well as those in which it is best to avoid it temporarily or permanently.

With this guide, therefore, you will be able to integrate intermittent fasting into your daily life, always taking into consideration our advice, your physical and health condition or the goal you hope to achieve with intermittent fasting. You must first remember that the beginning of any activity that requires getting used to something is going to be difficult, and intermittent fasting is no exception. Calming that 'phantom appetite' will take you a few weeks of adaptation, although when you control those cravings you will experience the multiple benefits of fasting for your health and figure. We invite you, therefore, not to give up, insist if you fail and go testing what kind of diet is best for you in practice. Through trial and error (always considering all relevant medical opinions when required) you will be able to find the intermittent fasting with which you can identify yourself in your daily life, making it as natural as any other activity. Good luck in the process!

Bibliography

Smith, J. (2019). *Intermittent Fasting 16-8: Lifestyle Guide*

Thompson, C. (2018). *The Art of Intermittent Fasting*

Fung, J. and Moore, J. (2017). *The Complete Guide of Fasting*

Vasquez, M. (2019). *The Guide to Intermittent Fasting and the Ketogenic Diet a*

Mosley, M. and Spencer, M. (2013). *The Fast Diet*

Legg, J. (2018). *Intermittent fasting*

I'd like to tell you how much Amazon ratings help me. Please rate this manual, and if it is possible, write your honest opinion about it. Comments help me improve and good reviews help increase the sales of this book, something that allows me to dedicate a little bit more time to writing. Thank you!

-   Damon Reed